WHY CAN'T A WOMAN BE MORE LIKE A MAN?

WHY CAN'T A WOMAN BE MORE LIKE A MAN?

A WOMAN'S GUIDE TO REVITALIZING HER NATURAL SEX DRIVE

MICHAEL P. BONAVENTURA, M.D.

THE SUMMIT PUBLISHING GROUP • ARLINGTON, TEXAS

THE SUMMIT PUBLISHING GROUP
One Arlington Centre, 1112 East Copeland Road, Fifth Floor
Arlington, Texas 76011

Printed in the United States of America
96 97 98 99 00 011 5 4 3 2 1

Library of Congress Cataloging-in-Publication Data
Bonaventura, Michael P. (Michael Patrick), 1952-
Why can't a woman be more like a man? : a woman's guide to revitalizing her natural sex drive / Michael P. Bonaventura.
p. cm.
ISBN 1-56530-184-6 (hard : alk. paper)
1. Women—Sexual behavior. 2. Sexual excitement. 3. Sex (Psychology)
HQ29.B66 1995
613.9'6—dc20 95-46867
CIP

Cover and book design by David Sims
Photography by Billy Stone

Table of Contents

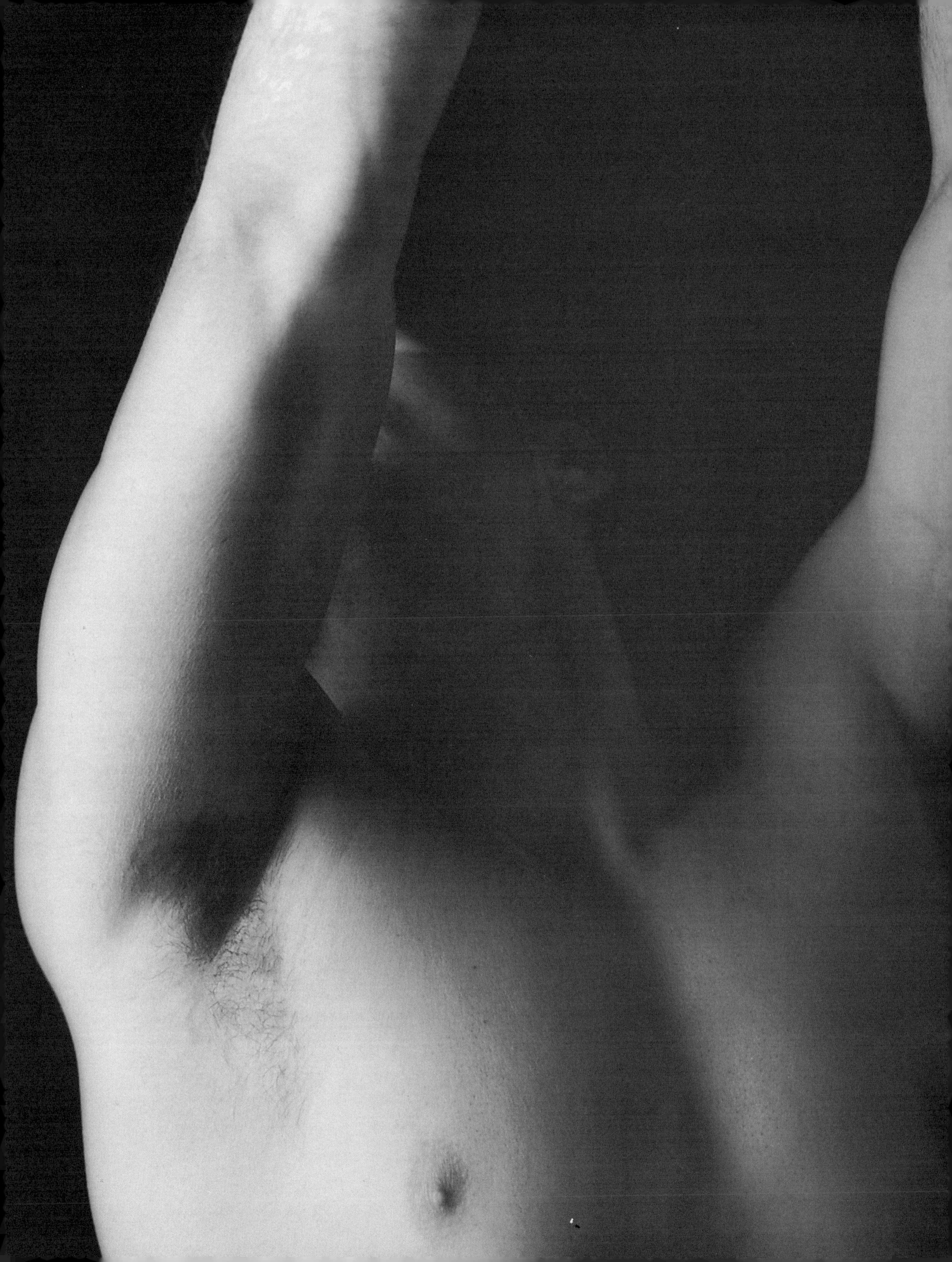

1

Chapter One

The Libido Gap

Today's woman lives in a world that has been shaped by many factors: the Sexual Revolution, women's liberation, sex education, legalized abortion, the "sharing, caring" male, colored condoms and the wonderbra®, Oprah and Phil, *Cosmopolitan* and the Pill, and, yes, cigarette ads that tell a woman that "You've come a long way, baby." On the surface, these factors would seem to promise her a golden age of sexuality.

But is it really golden? Or does today's woman still face issues that have not been addressed by advances such as the Sexual Revolution? For example, did the Sexual Revolution improve how women view their own sexuality? Did it improve how men and women treat each other? Did it rid them of their sexual hang-ups? Was there a revolution at all, and if so, who won? In short, have women really "come a long way"?

Not long enough, judging from what women tell me. Certainly not in the area of sexual equality. As a physician for thirteen years, I have listened to hundreds of female patients tell of their sexual frustration. Most often that frustration centers on the libido gap, that is, the difference between the lower sex drive of women and the higher sex drive of men. And, indeed, nearly every study of human sexuality confirms that the libido gap is real, that women do have a lower sex drive.

Why is there such a gap between the female and male libidos? This, to me, is the crux of the problem. Is the libido gap merely a matter of too much or too little testosterone? Could the problem be merely psychological? Could it be environmental or natural? Most important, does the problem have a solution?

My research reveals one undeniable fact: The libido gap is not natural. It is, quite literally, manmade—the product of centuries of sexism and socialization that have repressed the natural sex drive of women while condoning, if not encouraging, the sex drive of men. From childhood, women in our society are taught that being sexual—thinking about sex, talking about sex, much less *having* sex—is not something that a "good girl" does. This repression of a woman's natural sexuality creates guilt, conflict, and frustration for her and for the man in her life. This repression shrinks her libido, and as a result she has to overcome years of conditioning before she can "let go" and enjoy sex whenever she wants.

And the problem only worsens with time. Granted, at the start of a relationship, because sex is a natural urge in all people and because the initial novelty overrides a woman's conditioning, she may be able to rise above her repressive upbringing, stifle the nagging voices from her childhood, and express her natural sexual drive, which is just as robust as that of a man. But eventually she finds her sex life becoming routine and dull, as often happens in the average long-term relationship. Complacency sets in. That repressed upbringing comes creeping back.

One patient told me: "When we first started going out I couldn't wait until he came over. Every time I saw him all I wanted to do was have sex with him! I felt so sexy. Half the time he didn't know what hit him. But after several months had passed, he asked me why I didn't jump all over him anymore. I hadn't even noticed that things had changed. But he was right. Even though I thought he was still one hell of a sexy guy, things started to become more routine, and I wasn't as quick to get all 'hot and bothered.' I didn't know why!"

Couples who check out fine physically and who love each other come to my office for help, complaining of a huge libido gap. The man feels denied and increasingly resents the fact that the woman is seldom in the mood. And if the two of them do happen to connect, he resents the time that it takes her to respond. His attitude is, "The table is set; let's eat!" The woman resents the man's never-ending advances: "Doesn't he ever think of anything but sex?" she asks.

Her confidence in her sexuality takes a beating, and she begins either to fake orgasm or to resist sex altogether. She becomes increasingly bitter because he always wants to "fast forward"—sexually speaking—straight to the action scenes while she's still looking for the remote control. Instead of being flattered that he finds her desirable, she is angry because she can't keep up with his sex drive. After all, it's not as if she can force her body to speed up the arousal process. (Or can she?) She'd like to be more highly sexed, but that's not possible. (Or is it?)

Few relationships can survive such frustration.

For a relationship to work, men and women must be friends, not enemies. Instead of finding new ways to blame one another for sexual problems, we should focus on why these problems exist and *how to solve them.* Name-calling and blame-placing only aggravate an already strained relationship. Our goal should be to learn to understand and complement each other physically, emotionally, and sexually. In this way, sexual frustrations can become as extinct as dinosaurs.

At first, when patients approached me with concerns about the libido gap, I referred them to other doctors who were considered to be "experts" in sex therapy. "Sex therapy is not my specialty," I told my despondent patients. But most of them returned to my office expressing disappointment in the "experts." Common complaints included: "The doctor you sent me to just talked my problems to death, without offering any actual help" and "I need more than just talk… I need something to speed up my sexual metabolism."

It became clear to me that a new therapy is needed—a therapy that is based on common sense, simplicity, and a comprehensive knowledge of the physical and emotional facets of sexual relationships. So I developed Solid Therapy—a system of mental exercises, perfected through trial and error and the generous cooperation of my patients, that lets the female libido become spontaneous and less repressed. After all, if a repressed libido can be learned, it can be unlearned.

Using the exercises of Solid Therapy as the key, you can unlock the door to your natural sexuality. With the exercises as guides, you will learn to become more comfortable with erotic thoughts and more easily stimulated. You will be taught to center on your real-life experiences and erotic fantasies—things that really turn you on. You will learn to expand upon those experiences and fantasies to create ideal romantic scenes. Then you can become a camera and take mental "snapshots" of those scenes that especially arouse you. Those snapshots will be there for you to call up whenever you want. When you want to cut through the "red tape" of a repressed libido, you will pull a "snapshot" out of your mental photo album, and presto: instant desire!

Learning how to use personal thoughts to excite yourself will be your first step in Solid Therapy. It will also be your first challenge, because even under completely favorable circumstances many women find it difficult to initiate sexual thoughts. Unlike a man, a woman often blots out sexual stimuli. A woman will turn her eyes from erotic billboards, she will pretend not to notice a glistening male body parading on the beach, she will ignore the explicit song and avoid the X-rated video. She uses a sort of mental sunblock that shields her from the powerful sexual rays that bombard her every day. In a sense, she becomes her own sexual worst enemy.

The term *Solid Therapy* was selected after much consideration. I wanted to make it clear from the beginning that these mental exercises are not mere flights of fancy or vague "fluff" pretensions. Solid Therapy is just what it implies—therapy that is solid, concise, and specific. Just as physical exercises strengthen the body, so these mental exercises will strengthen your imagination and free the erotic potential buried within your psyche.

Solid Therapy will enable you to recognize the sexual stimuli around you and to use them to your advantage. As you become more comfortable with sexual feelings, you will be able to access these stimuli more quickly and able to become stimulated more easily. For instance, let's say that thirty minutes before you have to leave your home to eat out, you catch a glimpse of your significant other in the bathroom. He's shaving while wearing only a bath towel around his waist. Whereas before you were never one to initiate a "quickie," after Solid Therapy, you might well do just that—to the delight of you *and* him. That's just one of the benefits of my system.

Is the libido gap a widespread problem? While developing Solid Therapy I gave more than four hundred women a questionnaire about the variances in sexual desire between men and women. The responses indicated that virtually 100 percent of all relationships experience some degree of libido gap. And surveys, such as one conducted by Michael Kimmel of the State University of New York at Stony Brook, show that mature women, in increasing numbers, express dissatisfaction with their sex lives and partners.

This dissatisfaction is ironic in light of the chain of progress that twentieth century women supposedly have forged in their professional, political, and domestic equality. Let's take a closer look at what has been touted as one of the strongest links in that chain: the Sexual Revolution. During the late 1960s and early 1970s, you could not open a newspaper or magazine without reading about the latest sexual phenomenon and how it was going to change the world. The Sexual Revolution was going to change the way that men and women view sex and their own sensuality—make us all more at ease, more open, and more able to communicate our needs, our likes, and our dislikes to our partners as well as to ourselves. No more games. No more frustrations. The future promised an exciting, fulfilling sex life.

A generation later we are reminded about a multitude of sexual attitudes, from promiscuity to celibacy, that were influenced by the Sexual Revolution. But how much has really changed since then?

Let's look first at the postrevolutionary woman. We certainly can say that some things have changed for her. Girls, despite attempts at planned parenthood, are engaging in sex at an increasingly early age. Teenage pregnancy rates have increased at an alarming rate. Women are still ultimately responsible for birth control. The increase in rape figures is frightening, even without taking into account the number of women who are too afraid or embarrassed to come forward and become a statistic. Date rape and marital rape also make these figures swell.

Physical and emotional abuse of women and children is markedly on the upswing. Reports of sexual harassment in the workplace are up dramatically. The increase in exploitation of women in the media is evident: The blatant portrayals of women as nonintellectual sex objects are common on TV, in magazines, books, and movies. It has become so commonplace that some of the most offensive examples can be seen just by turning on MTV. Women are still regarded as inferior. That is evident even in our vernacular, with phrases such as "you son of a bitch" insulting women even when aimed at men.

In his book *The Glass Ceiling,* Bob Adams wrote that women still are paid less for comparable work and that, indeed, the number of meaningful jobs available to them has decreased to an unbelievably low level. The rate at which women are climbing the corporate ladder to meaningful positions has increased very little in the past twenty years. The glass ceiling remains as thick as a brick.

Now let's look at the postrevolutionary man. How changed is he? Too often he still wants to be the boss. He still balks at doing his share of the domestic chores. Yet when asked, a man has no trouble telling you what's wrong with his woman or with women in general. And he's not shy in voicing his unhappiness with how his needs and wants, especially the sexual ones, are being met.

The old adage that "men are after only one thing" still holds true all too often. Many men, apparently, are more interested in a shallow one-night stand rather than in a meaningful long-term relationship.

Men still don't seem to require love or emotional intimacy to engage in a satisfying sexual union. Many still have difficulty in being truly intimate with their sex partners and find it difficult to express honest emotion, no matter how long-standing a relationship becomes.

Our modern-day man, God bless him, may appear to be adaptable, to be willing at least to attempt to create a personal relationship by being the way his woman wants him to be: more sensitive, caring, and intimate. However, in most cases the makeover lasts only until the conquest has been made. In no time, he reverts to his old selfish self.

So, with all that, did the Sexual Revolution really take place? I find little evidence that it changed the attitudes and actions of men and women to any measurable degree. Indeed, I believe that the only result was that people had a little more sex but enjoyed it less! And if you ask me if the Sexual Revolution changed men, I would say that the facts suggest that while the revolution was going on, men were at home watching *Monday Night Football.*

Is there any hope for reforming the postrevolutionary man? The answer is, alas, "no."

For that reason, changing the sexual attitudes and behaviors of an emotionally uneducated thirty-year-old male isn't worth the effort. Expecting him to change is like expecting a leopard to change its spots. Besides, I have concluded that a man's sex drive is more natural than the culturally repressed woman's. Let's face it: Men, unlike women, have been conditioned to express, not repress, their sexuality.

Common sense tells us that it would be wiser—both psychologically and physically—to restore a woman's natural libido than to restrain a man's. Doesn't it make sense to teach women how to be sexually aggressive so that they can match men's intensity and rate of arousal? After all, sex is one area where a woman should be—and can be—the equal of any man.

In a perfect world, both partners would be equally involved in sex. But the world is far from perfect, and if the libido gap is going to be narrowed, it's up to women to do it. With Solid Therapy I am offering you a unique opportunity to improve the quality of life for yourself and future generations. Are you willing to face the challenge? With my program of exercises you can improve your love life by conditioning your mind and body—first by discovering what turns you on, then by learning to focus intensely on stimuli, and, finally, by teaching your body to respond to the images that you've selected.

You are unique, of course, and I have found that different stimuli work for different women. For instance, some women are excited by certain smells, others by the feel of silk, still others by music or a deep baritone voice. What excites one woman may turn off another or leave her indifferent. That's the beauty of Solid Therapy—it lets you create your own system to uncover your most erotic feelings, feel at ease with them, and make them accessible. Think of them as vitamin pills for your libido.

To master Solid Therapy, you will need to invest at least twenty minutes a day five days a week for seven weeks. Soon after, you will be able to look back and say, "Hey, I *have* come a long way!"

Before continuing to Chapter two, please answer the following questions candidly. Remember that there are no right or wrong answers—only answers that will help you to diagnose your problems and deal with them. Now get a pencil, relax, and let yourself go.

Does it take you much longer than your partner to "get in the mood" for love?

Yes - he's frustrated by this & I am as well.

Do you think your partner gets impatient waiting for you to become aroused?

Yes - he's confused as to why I am disinterested or why I resist -

If you can't slow down your partner's sexual desires, are you willing to "speed up" yours?

I don't feel I have a choice if I want my marriage to last

Do you agree that your relationship is important enough to work at and that you love your husband or significant other enough to implement change in yourself?

Yes - I'd like to create a more 'normal' & consistent existence for both of us.

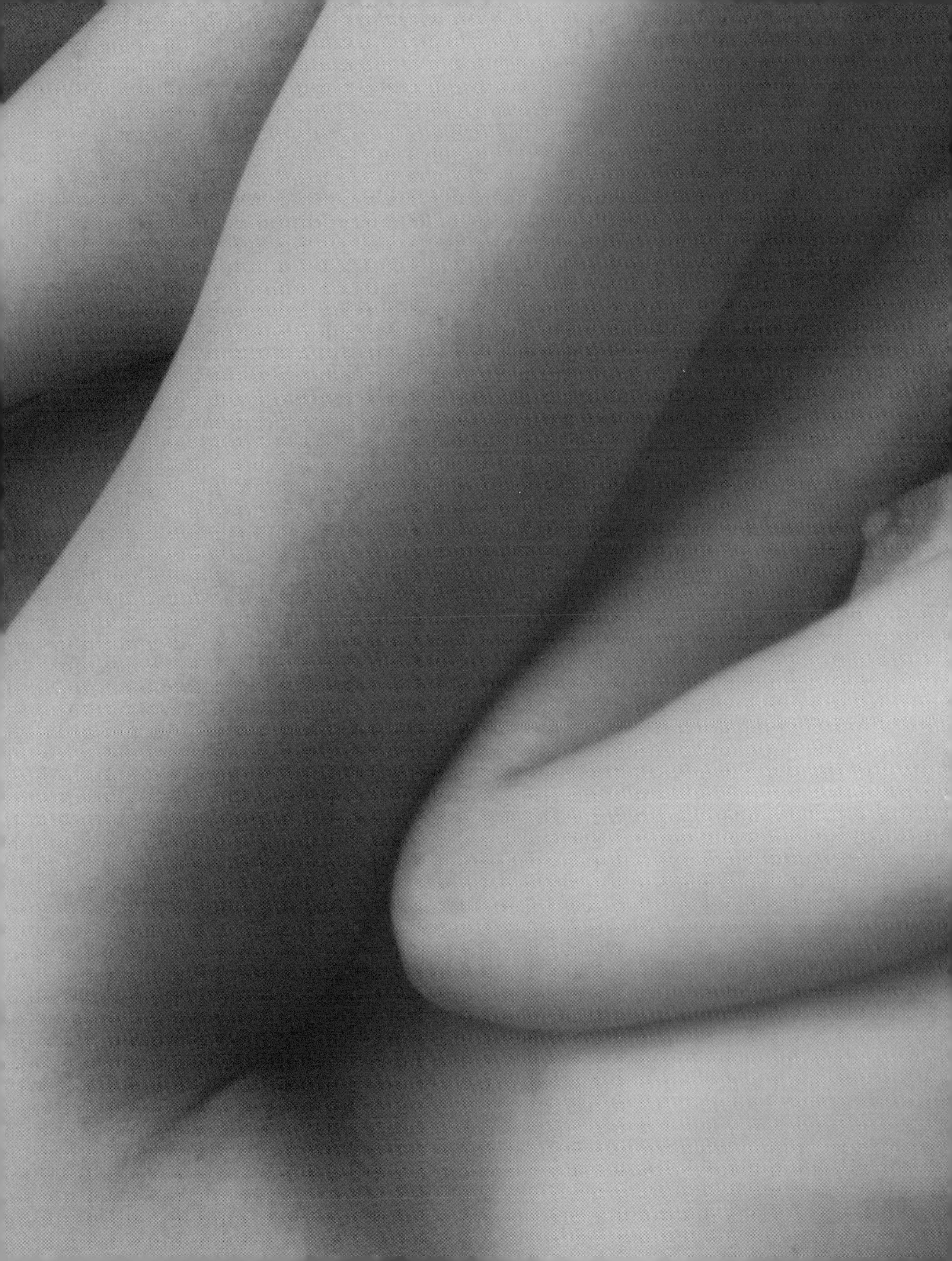

2

Chapter Two

Why Solid Therapy?

As April and Ryan entered my office, April burst into tears. "Ryan's going to divorce me," she sobbed. "He claims that I don't love him, that if I loved him, I'd be eager to make love with him like I used to when we first got married! He says it shouldn't take me so long to 'heat up.'"

April, an attractive thirty-four-year-old retail buyer, had been married to Ryan for seven years. The first two years had been happy enough, with both being quickly aroused and eager to please each other sexually. They seemed to be compatible. But then things began to change. Their lovemaking became less frequent and less satisfying. The problem was one that I had often seen in my practice. Ryan had a normal male sex drive, and April had been able to keep up with him sexually before they married and for almost three years after. But slowly, as the novelty of married life wore off, April's sex drive decreased to what most medical people consider to be a normal, less aggressive female libido. In simple terms, Ryan's libido remained stable, while April's plummeted and then leveled off. And herein lay the problem.

"By the time I'm finally ready to make love, he's either given up in frustration or fallen asleep," April complained. "I love him, I really do! I love having sex with him, too. I find him as exciting today as I did when we were making out before we got married. The problem is: It takes me a long time to push aside the cares of the day, and then we have to wait some more because it takes my body so damned long to respond to Ryan's lovemaking."

Ryan and April were considering divorce because of sexual incompatibility. Neither could satisfy the other. Whereas Ryan's sexual advances originally had ignited April's own passion, now she felt overwhelmed by sex. The more he pressed, the longer it took her to become aroused.

"If she were really interested, she'd still get excited about jumping into bed with me," Ryan declared, and then frowned. "There's no fire left in our relationship."

April, close to tears, blurted out, "I do love you, Ryan. It just takes me a long time to 'get excited.' I can't help it. Women just need more time to get aroused. I can't just click the remote on my sex drive and jump into bed! Why can't you just slow down and take your time? I'm tired of pretending to be excited," she wailed. "I want the real thing."

As I listened to April and Ryan, I thought of all the other patients who had come through my office with similar complaints. I again thought that this is not a race between the tortoise and the hare to see who gets aroused first, but rather a race in which the ideal outcome is a tie—when the two participants finish neck and neck. That way, they both win.

Women can't keep up with men mainly because their libidos have been artificially repressed. Thus they can't turn their thoughts from the mundane (job, bills, children, etc.) to the erotic as quickly as men can. "I'm a good wife, mother . . . Sex is my last priority," they seem to think. Is it any wonder they can't get aroused as quickly as men?

Today, because couples spend so much time and energy on family and career, and because AIDS and venereal diseases have caused people to curtail their sexual activities—or, at the very least, to limit the number of their sexual partners—they try to make every encounter more meaningful for both partners. Quality has replaced quantity. Thus it is more important than ever for a woman to concentrate on the satisfaction received from her sexual relationships.

Solid Therapy can help a woman achieve that satisfaction. Solid Therapy can teach you to accelerate your libido. By training yourself to focus on the details of mental images that are based on real or imagined erotic scenarios that *you* select, you can rediscover the sexual stimuli hidden in the people, things, and events in your life. And after you develop strong associations between those elements and your libido, you can widen your sensual associations to other once-neutral elements. The more elements you can associate with an erotic experience, the more erotic thoughts you will have and the quicker you will become aroused.

It doesn't matter whether you perceive these stimuli consciously or not, because it's the application of them that matters. If you become accustomed to associating sexual thoughts with a can of soda, afterward when you see a can of soda you will think of something sexual, and you will feel sexy.

Just as important, you will strengthen the mental pathways that connect such elements to erotic thought—strengthen them until they seem to be almost genetic. Imagine how opening hundreds of new erotic pathways will get the attention of your libido!

But first there are some ingrained attitudes to unlearn—attitudes that hamper your libido. Regardless of your level of sexuality, whether you are eighteen or eighty-one, you may become embarrassed when you think about sex. Oh, you may daydream a little, may enjoy fantasizing about foreplay, but usually the daydream or the fantasy stops just before the action starts! And if you allow your mind to go only so far and then apply your mental brakes, you may find yourself doing the same thing in real life: Everything is going along smoothly, when suddenly you hear a little voice shout "Stop!" All at once your mind, which has been doing seventy-five in an erogenous zone, screeches to a halt. Your body frantically says, "It's all right, it's all right," but years of conditioning say otherwise.

It takes a lot of coaxing from you and patience from your partner to silence that nasty little voice! That censor is a well-meaning mechanism, learned long ago, that was originally intended to protect you from harm. But now it becomes a nasty busybody, damaging your relationships and sabotaging your sexual satisfaction. Solid Therapy enables you to win over that troublesome little censor who always growls, "no, no, no" when more than anything you want it to coo, "yes, yes, yes."

It is important that women learn how to mentally "shift gears" from mundane to erotic thoughts. Many women have taught themselves to confine sex and sexual thoughts to a certain time and a certain place. Therefore, thinking about sex outside of these narrow parameters is foreign and uncomfortable. Again and again I hear: "It's a real chore to start thinking about sex" and "I get a funny feeling in my stomach just knowing that I'm going to start thinking about sex" and "It is so hard for me to just start thinking about sex. Once I do I really like it, but to get going I really do need a kick start."

In fact, thinking about sex outside of its "proper" time and place is so difficult for many women that they'd rather not even try. What a barrier to good sex that is!

One woman said: "When I started doing my [Solid Therapy] lessons it felt weird... especially during the day, it seemed strange, like it was at the wrong time and the wrong place. I could do it at home and at night without any problem, but during the day it was harder. Pretty soon, as time went on, it got much easier. Making yourself start at times when it felt unnatural was the toughest part."

With the help of Solid Therapy you can teach yourself to think about sex when you want to, to enjoy lust for what it is. Rather than feel guilty, you will become comfortable with yourself. In short, you can convince yourself that sex is healthy and enjoyable, not a sinful act that must be submitted to only after your defenses have been broken down.

Learning how to prepare yourself to think about sex is the most difficult element of Solid Therapy, but it is crucial to obtaining maximum results. In the beginning you may need to direct your thoughts consciously until you feel more comfortable doing so. If you are one of the lucky ones, this process will come easily, and you will enjoy the exercises that much sooner. Either way, it is important that you follow the exercises as they are laid out. I can tell you what to do and how, but in the end *you* have to *do it*.

It's important that you want to make your sex life better and to strengthen your libido. After you're motivated, it's just a matter of going through the written exercises and mastering the visualization techniques of Solid Therapy. You will soon find, as men do, that "getting there" is half the fun!

Such was the case with April, who found herself teetering with Ryan on the brink of divorce. Small wonder that she was eager to try Solid Therapy. She diligently read the materials I gave her, kept records of her experiences and fantasies, and eventually sketched them out in ever brighter and more colorful details. After she was confident that she could use her mind to arouse her body, she began the second stage of therapy, which consists of mental exercises scattered throughout the day, reinforcing the erotic images and giving her instant access to them. Within eight weeks, April could mentally "slip into something more comfortable" at will. She and Ryan were delighted with the difference that her renewed eagerness for sex made in their relationship.

I have found that women who graduate from Solid Therapy have a stronger libido and a feeling of greater self-confidence. Self-confidence is an amazing power! I've witnessed time and again the dramatic difference in people's personalities when they go from having little or no self-confidence to feeling good about themselves and confident about their abilities. It's incredible to see how an increase in self-confidence affecting one aspect of a woman's life so readily spills over into nearly every other sphere.

I'm not saying that when you complete my program you will experience an incredible surge of self-confidence in everything you do. But after guiding nearly one hundred women through Solid Therapy during three years, I can assure you that after completing this program you will feel better about yourself. And anything that can make people feel better about themselves has an amazing effect on their entire lives. Greater self-confidence leads to a more fulfilling love life.

Because I am not with you to answer all the questions you might have as you go through your therapy, I have included a questionnaire with answers from patients. These answers do not have to be *your* answers. They're just there to get you started—to gently illustrate some possibilities. Also, at the back of the book, beginning on page 159, is a Workbook Section which augments and reinforces the exercises. There are also interviews with several patients—interviews designed to answer nearly any question that you might have.

You also are provided with sample fantasies and memories of former patients. As you read them, think how you can apply their experiences to yourself. At the same time, ask yourself, "What do I like about sex? What excites me? What in particular about a certain man, or men in general, turns me on? Have I had a sexual experience that 'shook the earth'? What would it take for me to feel such passion?"

Remember: Don't hold back. Don't just romanticize. Eroticize!

Before we go to the next chapter, I would like to share the case of one patient.

Patricia had been skeptical of Solid Therapy. "It's too easy to be effective," she said. Patricia was a very intelligent woman, having graduated with a bachelor's degree in psychology, and had aspirations to enter graduate school. Although she wanted to increase her sexual desire, she did not believe that one's libido could be improved by a learned behavior or by therapy. But, because nothing else had worked, she decided to try Solid Therapy.

Although she experienced what she considered to be a slow start, she continued with her therapy. She often remarked: "This won't work for me. It will probably work only for someone with a weak personality…someone easily manipulated. It just won't work for someone who is intelligent and strong-willed."

Six weeks after her initial visit to my office, she called me. With a little irritation in her voice she told me that the day before she had been to a shopping mall. She had stopped in a store's fur department to try on a coat or two. By the time she left the store, she was beginning to feel turned on. When she reached home, she was "definitely in the mood." Her boyfriend walked in the door an hour later with plans for a movie and a late snack. Well, they never made it to the movie. Instead, they starred in their own form of adult entertainment and ended up ordering pizza afterward—three hours later!

"It wasn't until this morning," she said excitedly, "that I realized what had come over me yesterday. It was the furs!"

Patricia, who claimed she had no imagination whatsoever, had chosen for one of her Solid Therapy study aids a picture from a fashion magazine ad that she found very erotic. The ad depicted a very fashionable woman wearing a full-length fur coat in the foyer of what appeared to be an exclusive bar, waiting for someone. The coat was open just enough to reveal that aside from jewelry, stockings, a garter belt, and attractive underwear, the woman was wearing very little. The place was full of people, men and women, most of whom had noticed her with obvious appreciation.

"Whenever I think about furs, or stroke them," Patricia said, "I find myself getting worked up. Damn, it really worked!"

There may or may not be furs in Patricia's future, but it was pretty obvious that she had found a way to keep herself warm.

You may feel a little overwhelmed by all the material that you need to learn or by how complex and rigid Solid Therapy appears to be. I intentionally designed the therapy to be overly extensive, knowing that even if a woman completed only a fraction of the program, she would see improvement. But you will find that it's not that difficult to do and almost always becomes fun. Just because I've admitted this, don't feel that you don't have to follow the lessons. You will achieve much greater results if you complete the therapy as outlined.

Remember: Your sex drive needn't take any more time than his does to rev up. It's within your power to become anyone's sexual equal. So don't give up. Rome wasn't built in a day. And neither was a healthy libido.

Before proceeding, answer these questions as honestly and thoroughly as you can. Write your answers in the spaces provided.

How much time a day do you spend thinking about sex?

Very little most days; Occasionally there will be moments in days where I will fantasize; these thoughts will return fleetingly throughout the day.

Do you enjoy thinking about sex?

Yes - it's certainly pleasurable, especially at inappropriate times - it seems a very guilty pleasure for me -

Do you consider yourself sexy? Why or why not?

Yes - when I'm feeling good about myself - I'm attractive enough, have attractive breasts, & can be funny, am very intelligent - I feel sexy when I'm responded to -
No - when I'm feeling bad about myself or my appearance - there are definite weight issues that I struggle with -

Do you feel guilty when you think or fantasize about sex?

Not really - it doesn't happen terribly often - like I conveyed already - I find it a guilty pleasure, sort of a lark - a joke on the rest of the world who don't know what I'm thinking about

Would you like to become, sexually, as "quick" as your partner?

No - I would like to become "quicker" than I am - by that I mean willing & eager at least every week or two -

Our gaps are far too long & it is all my doing - I don't like that I am causing this, but I don't always feel guilty about it, just sad & let down by life.

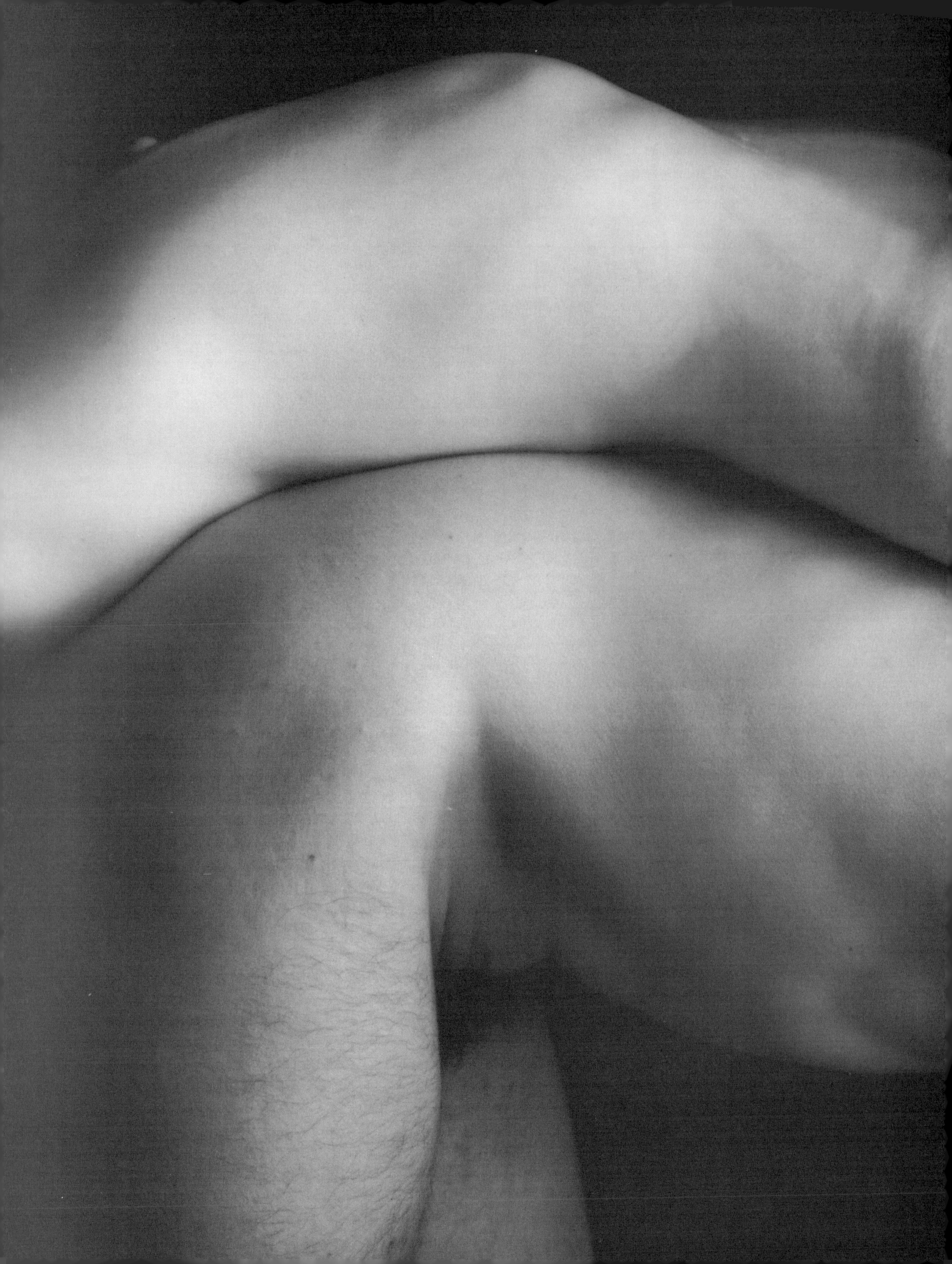

3

Chapter Three

Childhood: His and Hers

"My mom told me that sex is a dirty and disgusting thing...that should be saved for someone you love."

—a former patient

Before we begin your Solid Therapy, let's examine the early influences that family and society have on the sex drive of men and women. Let's see where we have come from so that we can see where we want to go.

Men and women are born with many things in common. We all need tenderness, intimacy, and nurturing. We all start life with eyes, noses, brains, genitals: All the equipment is there, beautifully designed, waiting for us to learn what it's for and how to use it.

But during childhood, boys and girls become trapped in a peculiar sexual apartheid that affects every aspect of their lives. If we can understand this apartheid and how it makes men's and women's libidos different, we can find a common ground for a better understanding of each other and improve the quality of our sex lives together.

Our first, and most important, influences are, of course, those frightened, well-intentioned (but frequently inept) adults whom we call "Mom" and "Dad." And of these two, Mom clearly is the bigger influence. In fact, according to *Psychology Today,* developmental child psychologists have found that more than 90 percent of what a child is exposed to is left up to the discretion of the mother or of the primary caregiver, who, again, is usually a woman. Research has shown that early impressions become central to our lives and become beliefs and habits that are nearly impossible to change.

Parental attitudes toward sex—informed or uninformed, healthy or unhealthy—govern what children learn, profoundly affecting the way that they view their own sexuality. Parents telegraph messages about sex to young children through both verbal and nonverbal conditioning. Although nonverbal conditioning remains important, as we become cognizant of our surroundings and learn language skills, verbal conditioning begins to play a more important role. Soon language skills become yet another weapon in a parent's arsenal—an arsenal that can be used to bestow a healthy upbringing or to inflict confusing and stifling messages.

Unfortunately, as infants grow into young children, parents seem to increase the confusing and sexist messages that they send about sexuality. Children have a natural curiosity about their environment, and they are no less curious about their own bodies. They may be even *more* curious about their own bodies because their bodies are usually all that they can get their hands on. It is only natural for children to be explorers.

Humans have sexual responses associated with genital manipulation as early as the first few weeks of life. These responses might not be classified as mature sexual responses, but they are observable nonetheless. It's at these early stages of life that sexual training begins, often riddled with repressive ignorance and prejudice. Many parents are uncomfortable with the fact that their children want to explore their genitals with as much interest as they do other parts of their bodies. Parents quickly caution their children that sexual organs are different and that children shouldn't treat them as they treat, for example, their noses or elbows. Therefore, children quickly learn that they are expected to confine such exploration to private moments and private places. It becomes something to hide, not to enjoy.

Children also show a natural curiosity about touching others and making comparisons. How many times has a child whom you are holding grabbed your nose, ears, or hair? The child is just comparing: "You've got ears, too!" And how many times have you heard a child innocently point out: "You've got a big nose"? You probably *don't* have a big nose, but from a child's perspective everything is larger.

So, too, children like to compare themselves with other children. Often they are mesmerized by each other, staring at and touching one another. This curiosity about others is shared by even the youngest child.

But if children are taught that it is taboo to explore their own "private parts," it follows that exploring someone else's body is just as taboo. Soon other feelings enter into an otherwise natural act: feelings such as guilt and the thrill of doing something they're not supposed to and the danger of getting caught.

As children grow old enough to verbalize their curiosity, their first questions concerning sex usually are directed to their parents. Those parents who can discuss sex with their children answer their questions with the misinformation and embarrassment that traditionally have been handed down from generation to generation, like distorted heirlooms.

Parents' uneasiness about their own sexuality greatly colors the way they handle their children's beginning awareness of sexual feelings. Children quickly learn that sex is a subject that parents would rather not discuss. The way that questions are answered or not answered speaks volumes to a child. Often a parent's uneasy manner lets a child know that sex is "dirty" or "secretive."

As children grow older, they have not only their parents to confuse them with sexual misconceptions, but also their peers and teachers.

But even though boys and girls have those misconceptions in common, the two genders are taught very different sets of rules and attitudes about sex. Boys are taught to be aggressive and to go after what they want. Boys are often encouraged to "sow their wild oats." They are expected to have sexual adventures with many partners. Strangely enough, this behavior is encouraged primarily by women: mothers, aunts, and so forth. How often have you heard mothers tell their sons: "Go out and play the field before you get married"? I've even heard a surprising number of women echo the traditional male advice to "Go out with lots of girls! You're too young to get tied down to just one yet! Why buy the cow when you can get the milk for free? You've got plenty of girls to go out with before you start thinking about settling down!"

When women see a cute little boy, they are apt to say: "Isn't he cute? Look at those long lashes. He's going to be such a *heartbreaker* when he grows up." But how often do people say of a cute little girl: "Isn't she cute? She's going to be such a *slut* when she grows up"?

This more "liberal" attitude creates fewer sexual hang-ups for boys. Boys are encouraged to explore and enjoy what comes naturally, without guilt, even if that means ignoring the feelings of others.

And yet despite being encouraged to play the field, boys are seldom taught how to please a woman. Many boys grow up not only as ignorant and inexperienced about sex as girls are, but also considerably more selfish. In fact, during the beginning of their sexual exploration, boys show very little concern about whether the girl is satisfied.

When those boys become men, society respects their feelings about their sexuality, which they wear on their chest like a medal for all to admire. Men who are considered great lovers are looked up to by nearly everyone. James Bond (007) is admired by both sexes for his sexual prowess, his animal magnetism, and his ability to have sex with one woman after another. He is licensed to kill *and* licensed to love.

Boys also can talk more freely about sex than girls can, and are allowed to learn at least the mechanics of sex more easily. Such interests are considered essential to a young man's development.

I have found that boys are often taught other bad behaviors—once again, curiously enough, by women. For example, they are taught that it's not a top priority for women to be smart, intelligent, and responsible. Boys also learn that it is more rewarding for males to be cool, rude, and aloof, and that sensitivity and stability aren't what women want. Although most women, if asked, will say they want a "nice guy," in reality "nice guys" finish last—they are the last ones chosen. Not many girls in school want to be seen with the "nerd"—the intelligent one who would probably wind up being responsible and dependable. Instead, I have found, they prefer the "bad boy"—the dangerous, insensitive one who has very few prospects for a stable future. Boys soon see that girls don't view intellect or responsibility as "cool."

Furthermore, women view a man who has had a good deal of "experience" in romance as desirable. And yet I wonder how much thought a woman gives to the other women who were hurt along the way by contributing to that man's "experience"?

Men have always had the upper hand when it comes to sexual satisfaction. Men don't blush about sex, agonize over it, or try to repress their feelings. The average man easily can daydream and fantasize about sex. It is not unusual for a man to think about sex thirty times a day and for almost everything to remind him of sex: a pretty girl, a whiff of perfume, a lingerie ad, a blank wall! With society's approval, he enjoys his sexual fantasies as well as memories of past sexual encounters and calls on "instant replay" to fill dull moments. He might find himself daydreaming and aroused at two in the afternoon, not realizing that his mind has made a subconscious connection between something from that moment and something from the past. Often he will go out with you, and bingo: All those pretty girls he's ogled, all those tantalizing whiffs of heady perfumes, all those lingerie ads tickle his libido. Suddenly all that energy is transferred to *you,* and *you* have become the immediate object of his desire.

What a different upbringing girls receive! Girls are taught to be passive, giving, nurturing…and vaguely ashamed about sex. It is amazing to see just how much sexual prejudice is involved in a girl's upbringing.

Let's first examine the prejudice in church dogma. Religion has a profound effect on how we view sex and, like other cultural influences, deals inconsistently with men and women. Church dogma is openly slanted toward the needs and wants of men. In church, women are taught that sex is meant to be pleasurable for men, practiced only for procreation, and that women should remain sexually pure and feel guilty if they have sexual yearnings. Apparently God gave women the ability to enjoy sex so that they could strengthen their character by denying their needs. I believe that the church's double standard can be explained in large part by the fact that men hold the positions of authority in most religions.

The conflict between learned morality and sexual reality is a source of conflict for many women. Many consciously repress their sexual feelings because they believe that sex is sinful. One woman said, "When I was a teenager, sometimes I would masturbate. But after I would climax I'd feel so wicked. I was taught that it was a sin to even think about things like that. I would feel so guilty that I would tell God I was sorry and promise I wouldn't do it again. But after a while I would start to feel horny again, and even though I would try to resist 'temptation,' I usually gave in."

The same double standard is taught in the home. Even in the most liberated of families, girls are cautioned about overt sexuality and told that because of their gender, liberties that are allowed to their brothers are strictly prohibited to them. This avalanche of prudery may convince a young girl that sex is dangerous and improper for her. Is it any wonder that most girls often find their natural curiosity about and desire for sex replaced with fear and sometimes outright aversion? Just as the ancient Chinese bound women's feet to keep them oppressed, so we have bound women's libidos to the past.

Girls, unlike boys, are taught to be sexually passive. In fact, society disapproves of a girl's being as sexually aggressive (promiscuous) as a boy. An experienced girl isn't looked upon with quite the admiration that an experienced boy is.

Because of this passivity, a girl is often confused as she seeks recognition and approval from others. As a result, she may feel embarrassed and insecure when dealing with her admirers. Unfortunately, she may drag these feelings along like a ball and chain the rest of her life.

Traditionally, girls have been taught—unlike boys—that sex should not be for their own enjoyment. Rather, girls are taught that sex is something to be shared and that one of their main goals is to make the man happy.

One woman said: "I was all set; I really thought I was in love with him. He led me to believe that he knew what he was doing. When we finally started, he just climbed on and climbed off, then left me lying there crying, thinking: God, this can't be all there is to it."

She continued: "I was so concerned that I wouldn't be experienced enough to satisfy him. That jerk didn't even care two cents about me."

Physical beauty is another trait that is stressed throughout a woman's life. This concern with beauty, like many other acquired attitudes, develops almost from birth. For a little girl, being pretty is a big plus. However, wanting to be pretty can cause confusion, and *being* pretty can cause resentment. For example, an eight-year-old girl comes downstairs dressed up in her mom's clothes, complete with high heels and makeup. Dad runs to get the camera to take her picture. Even though her lipstick goes up to her eyebrows, Dad beams, "She's beautiful." As Dad takes her picture she is told how pretty she is and how grown-up she looks. But take the same little girl at age fourteen. She's getting ready to go out with friends. She dresses up, fixes her hair, and puts on a little makeup. She's almost out the door when Dad says: "Where the hell do you think you're going dressed like that? Go upstairs and take that stuff off!" Being attractive to Daddy is fine, but after other males begin to notice, how attitudes change!

Girls are exposed to so many different signals about looks that often they don't know whether being pretty is a blessing or a curse. Of course, it can be both. An attractive young girl's parents may react negatively to the attention she receives, and friends may become jealous of it. She finds that being pretty even can be dangerous in certain situations. And a girl feels that if she's not as pretty as she would like to be, she might not get the type of attention she wants. In any case, appearance ultimately affects her personality development.

Even in dealing with their peers, girls not only must worry about not being "pretty" enough, but also often must worry about being too pretty and thus being the object of jealousy and alienation.

"We grew up together," one woman said. "We were best friends. Somewhere along the way she filled out more than I did and started getting all the attention! God! All the boys were crazy over her. It was like I wasn't around when she was there. I hated her for that. We were never close again."

The woman went on to say, "At times when I think about it, I still hate her for it."

Parents teach little girls to feel anxious about their bodies. Peers and society at large give them the same message as they grow up. It is obvious how dependent upon looks women have become in order to have a healthy self-image. In his book *Sexual Images of the Self* Seymore Fisher White wrote that more than 90 percent of all women are dissatisfied with their bodies and, if they could, would trade them for a better model. For example: "I think I've got great breasts, but I'd really like to trade in my thighs and butt."

Because the world remains male-dominated and the male perspective is still an overwhelming cultural influence, as girls grow up, that male perspective colors how they view their bodies and sexuality. When a little girl picks up a Barbie doll, she can easily see that Barbie doesn't measure five-foot-one and 32AA. When a girl watches women on television or in the movies, those women usually are beautiful, blond, and built.

To those who say that conditions are better nowadays and that women are no longer being held to those stupid old standards, I say this: "You're wrong!" And to those who say that the pressures on men are just as great, I say: "Wrong again!" It is still a one-sided problem. Men are far less discontent with their physical appearance than women are. Moreover, what discontent there is for men is far less intense than that for women. Men also state that "looks" are one of their most important considerations in choosing a mate. For women, "looks" are far less important. I believe this is one of the reasons why the number of plastic surgeries performed on women has increased 270 percent in the last five years.

Ignorance, hearsay, and hang-ups play a principal part in how most of us view and understand the workings of the female body. When a little girl's hand wanders to her genitals, a parent's first response usually is to prevent exploration. I've heard so many times, even from seemingly intelligent health care professionals, that if a girl touches herself "down there" she runs a higher risk of infections. As one of my patients stated, "Her hands might be dirty, and if I let her touch herself on her vagina she'll probably wind up with a bug, fungus, or yeast infection like I get all the time."

Preventing girls from touching themselves sends them the message that it's not "good" to touch themselves. They learn apprehension, and eventually this apprehension influences how they view themselves physically and sexually.

For example, one patient told me, "I feel funny when I see her [daughter] touch herself. It makes me feel weird. I think that if I let her do it, she'll just want to keep doing it more and more. And when she gets older, she'll probably start having sex at ten or eleven. So I figure I'll try and slow things up now, before they get out of hand."

Most women, when asked about childhood recollections, distinctly remember their inability to discuss sex with their parents. Many recall vividly those earliest such encounters. One woman said: "I was talking with other kids in the neighborhood about how babies were made. I was only about seven or eight then. I remember when I asked my dad about making babies. He stopped what he was doing, got a little fidgety, and said very fast, 'Ask your mother,' then left the room. Before I got a chance to ask my mother, my father went into the kitchen, and I could hear my mom and dad discussing the subject and what they should tell me about it. I remember it was the first time I heard the word *sex*. Even though at the time I didn't know what the word meant, I knew it caused a lot of commotion. I can still remember hearing my mother telling my father, 'She is too young to understand that stuff yet. I don't know what to say, either. Let's leave it alone; she'll probably forget all about it and go out and play.'"

She recalled her father's solution to the problem: "Keep her away from those little perverts."

That woman said that she was never able to discuss sex with her parents again. Even as an adult with kids of her own, she would always feel uneasy when the subject came up in the presence of her parents.

One patient said, "My little girl came up to me and asked me what a penis was. I was really shocked to hear her ask that. I kind of snapped at her and asked her where she heard that word. I could tell at once by the look on her face that my response scared her. She told me she had seen the word while looking through another child's book about sex. I couldn't think of what to say, so I just told her that I'd get her one of those books, too. She simply said OK and left the room. I was taken off guard! Afterward I realized I should have handled it differently."

The patient told me that even though she wanted to bring up the subject of sex again with her daughter, she never did. And she never bought the book, either, expressing the belief that it wasn't a proper way to handle the subject.

These are just a few examples of girls' first encounters with their parents' attitudes toward sex. Unfortunately, these examples are all too typical, due either to the lack of parental courage in confronting the issue or to the lack of easy access to qualified counselors, therapists, agencies, and written materials.

Unlike boys, girls are not able to talk as freely about sex and to learn at least the mechanics of sex easily. Girls fear that they might be viewed as trampy or might incur the disapproval of friends and parents if they show too much interest. Girls aren't supposed to be eager to learn about sex. As a result, most women keep their curiosity about sex a secret and do not develop a healthy knowledge of the "fun" side of sex.

Most information about sex doesn't come from parents but rather from peers. As we all know from our own experience, information disseminated by our well-intentioned friends is often long on fancy and short on fact. When consulting with friends, girls do far more talking about romance and less about sex, which is just the opposite of what boys do. It isn't considered "ladylike" for girls to talk about sex.

As one woman put it: "I wanted to know stuff about sex but was afraid to ask even my best friend, Mary. I felt embarrassed about it. I didn't want her to think I was bad or dirty for thinking about that kind of stuff. I always hoped she would bring up the subject, but she never did. I certainly couldn't talk to my parents."

Many women have stated that as girls they would try to find such information in their local libraries. I have visited several local public and junior high libraries, and what I found wasn't surprising: Very little material was available, and what was available was mostly too antiseptic, confusing, or difficult for a novice to understand. For example, Jane said, "I remember when I first heard the word *screw*, I really didn't have anyone to ask about it, so I tried to look it up. There were so many different definitions for it that I had no idea what was right...for the longest time I thought it meant to twist or turn. Once I tried to look up the word *boobs*. Boy, did I ever feel stupid when I found out what it really meant."

Jane shouldn't have felt stupid. Sex has a "casual" language that can't be taught in library settings.

Even good information about a fact as basic as menstruation is difficult to find. Parents often don't want to talk about it. Most women learn about "periods" from that great, all-knowing source of knowledge: their friends! What's even more tragic is that when there *is* good communication between parents and daughters, most parents themselves often don't understand the physiology of the menstrual cycle and end up causing more confusion than clarification.

A woman told me: "I was twelve years old when I had my first period...I thought I hurt myself while playing. I ran to my dad and he got mad at me and told me to 'go see your mother.' My mom told me that this is what happens when a girl turns into a woman. I was never aware that anything like that happened...it was quite a shock. She told me how to take care of it, but when I asked her why there was blood, she just told me that's part of what happens."

Eventually, the woman told me, she made a point of learning all there is to know about menstruation. However, when I asked her to be more specific, she answered: "I really don't understand it in that much detail."

Not only are many women ignorant about the subject, but they also view this perfectly natural occurrence as something dirty—a view that is another vestige of long ago. A woman said: "Way before I got my first period, a girlfriend of mine told me about the 'curse.' That it happens every month, hurts real bad, and guys think it's disgusting. Also I was going to have to start to worry about getting pregnant, couldn't go swimming at that time, and become weak from loss of blood."

Traditionally, girls have had to walk a fine line between being themselves and being what other people wanted them to be. Girls have to worry about what other girls, including friends, thought of them. If a girl doesn't seem interested in sex or doesn't act as if she knows much about it, her friends might consider her immature. But if she shows too much interest in sex, she might be thought of as "loose" or "slutty." Heads you lose, tails you lose.

Most women recollect early discussions about sex with their friends as a lot of talking and giggling, tossing out new words, slang, and questions, and then listening to the reactions. However, as we all know, kids can often be unkind to one another, and first impressions are often lasting ones:

"There were four of us; we were all about fourteen and were spending the night at Nancy's. All of us were laughing and talking about sex and things. I had previously heard some things about oral sex, and, well, it sounded pretty good to me. I wanted to tell them about it, but before I had a chance Mary said something about it. Right away she and Nancy both started to say things like 'Ewww, that's gross!' and 'Yuck, that's awful! The only people who do things like that are prostitutes and sluts like Sherry.' Sherry was a girl in our class who had a reputation for being 'loose.' Well, after a lot of 'ewww's and 'yuck's, I didn't want the others to think I was a whore or anything, so I didn't say a word about it. I'm convinced that after all this time my mixed feelings about oral sex came from that night. It's exciting to think about actually doing it. But there's fear that maybe they were right: Only whores and sluts do things like that. And I wind up feeling guilty because I like it."

Another major concern of girls, of course, is what boys think of them. When a girl is with her boyfriend, she worries about whether he can be trusted to be discreet. She agonizes: "Will my boyfriend keep our activities a secret, or will he be exaggerating in the locker room to all his friends, and ruin my reputation?"

To add to her misery, a girl worries that if she doesn't give in and "put out," she might be labeled a tease, stuck-up, or frigid. Conversely, if she goes all the way, will the boy respect her afterward? Even in this day, many men express a desire for a virgin and would never consider taking one of those "other kind" home to Mother.

Sometimes a girl starts having sex either to "prove" her love for her boyfriend or because she simply runs out of excuses and becomes exhausted by all the pressures. She often finds it easier to give in than to fight on. Boys have a wonderfully powerful line: "You got me worked up. It's your fault."

Many times a girl is made to feel guilty. One woman said: "We were dating for quite a while. I would frustrate that poor guy all the time. Finally I just felt so bad for him that I did it…for him! To top it all off, I felt guilty afterwards. I kept thinking that I was 'bad' for doing it. I kept wondering if he thought of me differently now. And whether or not he would still marry me, now that he had gotten what he wanted."

Another woman said: "I remember when I 'did it,' we were in his car after going to the movies. Things were getting pretty heated. I was always able to keep things pretty well in control. But I can still see his face. I felt so sorry for him. We had been through this so many times, and he always was so nice about it. So that night I figured he deserved it. It wasn't where I always thought my first time would be but …"

How many of you can recall the first time you had sex? Whether it was a good or a bad experience, the first time we have sex will leave an impression on us that can affect our adult lives. Unfortunately, most girls do not rate their first sexual experience as a good one.

For example, one woman said: "The first time I ever had sex was a mess; everybody had filled my head with so much junk. I was so worried about it before it happened. When we were finally doing it I was so darn nervous that I couldn't relax and enjoy anything."

A girl may be more concerned about whether she is "performing correctly": "Am I moving my body right? Am I making too much noise? Am I not loud enough? Will it hurt? Am I sexy enough for him, or will he be thinking of someone else? Am I making it good for him?"

This is because girls seem to have been better "trained" to please others than themselves and are better at giving than at receiving. When it comes to sex, the same seems to be true for them. A girl is supposed to know intuitively what a man wants and to supply it. Many girls are told that sex wasn't invented for their pleasure and that even if it were, their pleasure should wait until after the man is satisfied.

A girl's first experience is just one of the factors that reinforces a woman's tenuous libido. Why should she want to have sex four or five times a week when she doesn't enjoy it? Why should she let herself get sexually aroused, only to have her desire extinguished and to be left unsatisfied? It takes a tremendous amount of care, patience, and understanding on the part of her male partner to change such preconditioned sentiments. Better that a woman change herself!

In *Women and Love: A Cultural Revolution in Progress* Shere Hite wrote that women—single and married—expressed an increasing dissatisfaction with sex. And the duration of the relationship was not a factor. Whether it was a long-standing relationship or just a one-night stand, women were not deriving pleasure from sex and did not view it as a comfortable or wonderful experience.

Is this any surprise? After years of turning sexual feelings on and off, girls are supposed to emerge miraculously as passionate women when a legitimate adult situation, such as marriage, materializes. Ridiculous! Because a girl has practiced so hard at being readily able to turn off her feelings, it becomes physically and emotionally impossible—without serious relearning—for her to become a passionate woman who enjoys sex easily. It isn't easy for an anxious, uptight, in-control woman to ignore all of the negative conditioning from her childhood and all at once to release the floodgates and drown in sexual ecstasy.

Solid Therapy can help a woman to overcome that conditioning. And it has these advantages: Because it's a self-help program, you can complete the therapy in private and never be embarrassed by having to seek help in person. It's also inexpensive. And it's convenient. After all, by means of this book, your doctor makes house calls.

Before we move on, answer a few more questions. Take your time and be honest.

How did you find out about the "facts of life"?

How do you wish you'd been brought up regarding sex?

Does your religious background help or handicap you in a sexual relationship?

Can you recall instances as a child when you were warned that sex is bad or dirty or sinful?

Can you remember how you felt as an adolescent when you fantasized about love?

Did your first sexual encounter live up to your romantic dreams?

Do you think boys are "trained" to feel that sex is enjoyable and that their bodies are vessels of joy?

What sort of messages about sex do you send to your children? Do you plan to make your daughter(s) feel good about sex and, if so, how?

As a child, did you want to grow up to be smart or beautiful?

Did you feel satisfied with your body after it began to develop?

Do you think you have to be physically "perfect" to be a good lover?

How can you improve your self-image?

Do you think that Solid Therapy can help you get excited about love?

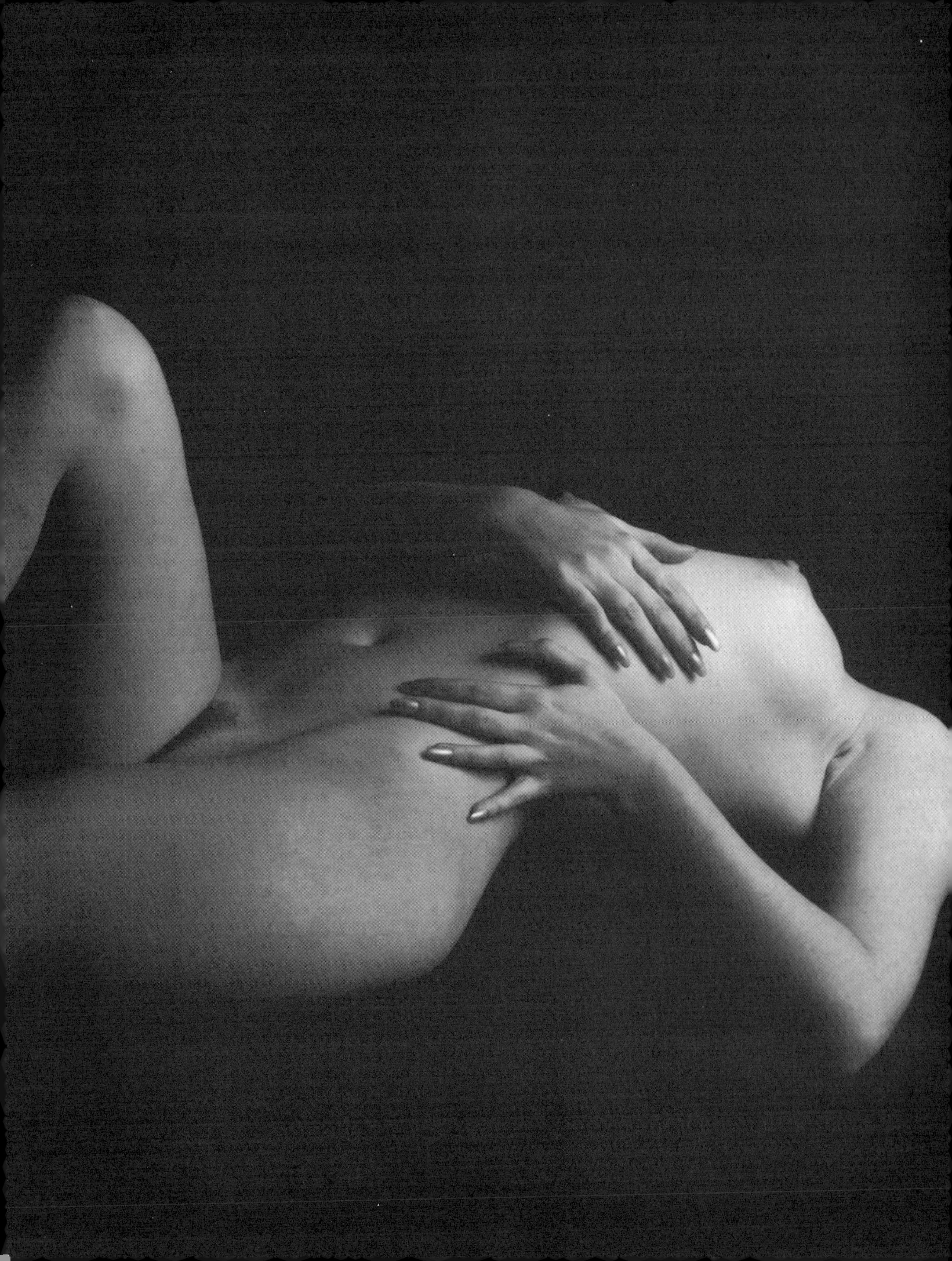

4

Chapter Four

Let Me Ask You This

A recent survey reported in *The CQ Researcher* found that some people have a greater number of sexual thoughts and daydreams than the average population does. According to the survey, these fortunate people are those who have weak religious ties, those women who as children had close emotional relationships with their fathers, those who have had rich sex lives, and those who generally have a more liberal attitude toward sex. It was found that not only do these people have a greater number of sexual thoughts and daydreams, but also that their thoughts and daydreams are longer, richer, and more explicit.

This survey also revealed that an individual's sexual thoughts, memories, and fantasies are more exciting and capable of evoking a significantly higher level of arousal than are other types of nonphysical stimulation, that is, watching explicit movies, reading romantic novels, and so forth.

No surprise there. I, too, have found that the time needed for people to become aroused is significantly lessened when they use a personal memory or thought instead of nonpersonal material.

This chapter is about what arouses you. There are several questions for you to answer in the spaces provided. Don't be afraid to "let loose" on paper. The more explicit you can be, the more aroused you can become as you go through Solid Therapy. Keep in mind that your work in this book is for your eyes only (unless you choose to share it).

With each question, search your mind and examine past experiences. I want you to write down those things that first come to mind as stimulating. But don't stop there. Although those first remembrances are most important, see if you can remember others that once aroused you but that you may have forgotten. Do not exclude anything that elicits an erotic or sensual feeling.

Accompany each of your answers with an explanation of why that particular response elicits erotic or sensual feelings in you. It is important that you write down your answers and not merely answer the questions in your head. This will enable you to imprint the necessary details firmly in your mind. If you are unsure how best to answer each question, review the examples. Take your time and be sure you follow the instructions as closely as possible. Again, I stress, this is a free-form exercise, not an essay contest. Write what you feel the way you feel it. Express yourself in the manner that is most comfortable to you.

Each of the questions is accompanied by several examples of how other people have answered them. Look over all the examples in each group after writing down your own answers. As you read through the sample answers, you will notice that some are much longer than others. This is entirely normal. Some respondents have more to say or enjoy elaborating, while others prefer to be more concise.

QUESTIONNAIRE

BODY

What part of a man's body turns you on? Are there one or more areas of your ideal man's body that excite you?

Focusing on the male (or female) body is a good tool for some women to help them release their inhibitions. Close your eyes and picture a male body, dressed or undressed. Play around with your mental picture. Make him blond or dark haired, tall or short, muscular or long and lean. Picture his eyes as brown or blue or hazel. If you find several areas that arouse you, list them in order of preference. Then write down whatever comes to mind when you think about each answer.

Everyone has preferences in bodies: Some women are "chest nuts," while others might like eyes, hair, lips, arms, legs, shoulders, fingers, and so forth. Remember that there are no right or wrong answers. We are trying to find out what arouses you, so give the answers some thought and be honest with yourself.

1. ______________________________

____

____

____

____

____

2.

3.

Here are some sample answers from other women:

1. **Eyes:** "What I like most in a man is his eyes. Give me a good set of baby blues to look at anytime…I mean, I just melt when my boyfriend looks deep into my eyes."

   Many women, however, will admit that more intimate body parts catch their eye.

2. **Butts:** "I am definitely a butt woman. I can be working or busy doing something and if a great butt walks by, I'll notice it right away. It's like I have great peripheral vision when it comes to that. I love men in tight bicycle pants. I won't be thinking about it, yet let one come into my range of vision and my eyes will lock on to it…I just go crazy at the beach in the summer."
3. **Smiles:** "I never really noticed smiles before. But there was this guy at work; he really wasn't that handsome, but when he smiled it would light up a room. He had the sexiest smile I had ever seen. He had nice lips and the whitest teeth. I couldn't get that smile out of my head. I just had to find out if it kissed as good as it looked. And did it ever! It sounds stupid, but I was seduced by a smile."
4. **Chests:** "A whole bunch of us from school were goofing off at a friend's farm. Luke and I had a crush on each other. We wandered off behind this old rundown barn. It was really hot that day. He was wearing a white button-down cotton shirt, and due to the heat

he had undone most of the buttons to try and cool off. As we stood next to each other I remembered thinking that I had seen his chest on several occasions before but never this close, close enough to touch. We were kissing for a while when I pulled away from him. He thought he was going a little too fast, but really all I wanted to do was to get another look at his beautiful chest. And it was beautiful; I really couldn't resist any longer; I reached out and touched it. I can still picture how my fingers looked as they moved over his skin; it was like they weren't mine. Then without thinking what I was doing, I knew I had to touch it with my face. I lowered my head and let my cheek lightly brush against his chest. It looked and felt so wonderful—tan, soft, and so smooth. I've seen some really nice ones since then, and whenever I see a man in a white cotton shirt, I always want to go right up to him, unbutton it, and check him out. But if you want to talk about standards, for me Luke's chest was…well, what can I say?"

Many women find a woman's body erotic as well. A woman can appreciate another woman's body as an object of beauty and desire without being a lesbian. Since ancient times, a woman's body has been looked upon as beautiful and artistic. In nearly every culture it has become universally revered by men and women alike.

5. **Breasts:** "I think boobs are attractive. When I see a woman with nice breasts, proportioned well, I find that attractive, especially if she isn't wearing a bra and has on a nice-fitting blouse. That's erotic. I love to look at women's lingerie ads."

SIGHT

Are there particular sights that elicit your sensual feelings?

Although sight may seem to be the most obviously sensual sense, this question is much more complicated than it appears because of the massive amount of visual stimuli that we are exposed to daily. Picking just a few sights from that constant bombardment may be difficult at first.

I had found that you have basically two types of visual stimuli: One comes from real-life experiences, that is, a handsome man catching your eye, and so forth, and the second comes from pictured material, that is, books, photographs, artworks, movies, and so forth. During my interviews with patients, many women stated they were not all that visually oriented, meaning that they didn't respond to visual material as strongly as men do. However, after examining what, if any, visual stimuli they might indeed find exciting, I concluded that they were right: Women aren't as visually oriented as men are. *They are more so!* The problem is with the perception of what is exciting to view.

Today, our societal and sensual norms are expressed from a man's point of view. There is ample evidence all around us that the male perspective is an overwhelming influence. Realizing this, it can be easily understood how a woman might feel that she is not as visually stimulated as a man is, considering that what *he* finds arousing is viewed as the standard.

When women said they didn't consider themselves to be "visual," their answer seemed to be influenced by the male point of view. And yet women can perceive more material as exciting than men are. (Smart advertisers have been aware of this for a long time and have been making women subconsciously feel good by projecting sensual feelings onto their products.) Not only can women at times find explicit materials arousing, but they also can view a variety of other materials as arousing and pull out subtle undertones, some of which are not outwardly viewed as erotic.

Sight is so important that it will be dealt with in more detail in Chapter Eight. Meanwhile, write down examples of visuals that stimulate you, and include an explanation or a description of your thoughts.

1. ______________________________

2. ______________________________

3. ______________________________

Here are some examples:

1. **A Well-Dressed Man:** "When I see a man all dressed up in a nice suit, white shirt and tie, that turns me on…I get visions of dinner, dancing, and a wonderful evening."
2. **A Uniform:** "I know it's the oldest cliché in the book, but when I see a man in a uniform, whether he's a fireman, a sailor, or an airline pilot, I just go berserk. Sometimes I tease my husband and tell him that the only reason I married him was because of his uniform (he's a policeman)."
3. **Tight Blue Jeans:** "I love it when a guy is dressed real casual, not out to impress me, and he's filling out his jeans, you know what I mean. That gets me really excited."

   Some women prefer to use a different form of visual eroticism. They use pictures from magazines or books:
4. **Muscles:** "A man with muscles turns me on. I look at those magazines for bodybuilders …the ones where the men stand around in tight trunks and flex their bodies and strike all those great poses. I know some of my friends think these men are gross, but the size of their arms and chests makes me feel so tiny and feminine in comparison! And I can just imagine being hugged by one of those muscle-bound Michelangelos."
5. **Half-Nude Men:** "I like pictures of men bare from the waist up…rugged types with jeans on. I must have a half dozen similar pictures in my locker and around my desk …chests, arms, and unshaven. I love to see a nice-looking guy in real life or in a magazine when he has about three days' growth on his face. I think of being in some cabin with him on a warm summer day."
6. **Snow and Cloudy Days:** "Well, I married him in spite of my reservations, thinking that things would eventually get better. However, even after trying to change things for nine years, I was never able to ignite any passion in him. And even though he had become very successful in business and we had everything we could ask for, life had become 'lifeless.' Finally, I couldn't go through the motions anymore. I needed to feel alive again. So, in spite of everyone's advice, I left him.

   "It was then that things became curious. It seemed that my leaving sparked, for the first time, some real emotion in him. He said he was sorry for being so expressionless all this time and that he understood my need for excitement and passion to be a part of our lives. And since he now realized all the cold and awful things he had been doing to me …to *us*…that he wanted to be different and that he deeply loved me. Well, I wasn't sure whether or not to believe him, but after watching the way he was reacting, and listening to him say things I had never heard him say before, I decided he was genuinely sincere and would give it a second chance.

   "We decided that if we were to try again, things had to be different. We would make sure that they would never again become boring or complacent. We'd find more time for ourselves, 'better' time for ourselves, and talk to each other. It was during this time that I had this experience.

"It was a typical afternoon in Chicago: gray and windy. I told my husband I'd pick him up from work a little early that Friday and we'd go check out a new restaurant that was supposed to be really romantic. It was about 3:45 P.M. when I pulled up in front of his office, which was located on a quiet little tree-lined street. The front of his building was done in dark brown bricks, large picture windows with white wooden frames, and forest green canvas awnings. The first floor and windows rise up about three feet above the sidewalk.

"From where I was parked I could easily see into the offices facing the street. As I was waiting, it began to snow. It wasn't like a blizzard, all blustery and nasty, but really beautiful. The snow fell slowly, with large heavy flakes. It made you feel close and safe, like you were being covered with a fluffy comforter. Mesmerized, I watched these beautiful creatures land all around me and begin to cover me in. My eyes slowly began to focus on a nicely dressed man in one of the offices. Because of the dark gray sky, the lights in all the offices appeared brighter than usual, and everything was quite visible, even through the snow. When I turned my wipers on to get a better look at this 'vision,' I realized the person that caught my attention was my husband! I had to chuckle to myself. I couldn't win…Here I was trying to scope out this good-looking guy, and it turned out to be the man I was married to. As I sat there watching through my windshield I began to feel funny.

"I had never seen him in this light before—at work, unaware and unaffected by my presence. I began to realize he was really a handsome man. His jacket was hung over the back of his chair and his white shirtsleeves were rolled up. The more I watched, the more I became mesmerized by him, becoming only slightly aware of the beautiful snow around me. He would walk about his office, talking to this one or that one, handing papers to his secretary while discussing 'important things' on the phone. The whole scene really did something to me. It was like I was seeing this man for the first time. I loved the way he looked and acted, not being influenced by my presence. And the more I watched him, the more excited I got. Excited to think that this powerful, handsome man was really mine! Mine to do with as I liked. I got so worked up that by the time he finally came out, I literally jumped all over him!

"For weeks after that day I couldn't keep my hands off him. For me it was like we were newlyweds all over again.

"I always get warm and erotic feeling whenever I see an old office building, heavily overcast days or snow. I really can't control my feeling when I do."

7. **Roller Coasters — Amusement Parks:** "It was the summer between my junior and senior year in high school, when a large group of us decided to go to Great America [theme park] for the day. We were all from the same school and knew each other. I had a crush on this one guy there, 'Kevin,' who was about the biggest hunk in school. Back then I thought I was pretty cool myself, having been a cheerleader for three years and

quite popular with both the guys and girls. But for some reason he never seemed interested in me. Even though he was really hot and nearly every girl in school wanted him, it didn't go to his head. He was really sweet and quiet. I guess you would call him shy.

"A couple of days before the outing, Kevin called and asked me if I was going to be there; he said he wanted to talk to me about something. I kind of had a hunch he wanted to ask me out but was too afraid. That day was pretty warm so I decided to wear loose-fitting clothes to help stay cool: a white cotton short-sleeve pullover shirt and large, tan, baggy, safari shorts (and no underwear).

"Everyone was having a great time with all the rides and eating everything in sight. But I was doing even better! Kevin had been taking every chance to get close to me. And when we would talk, I could tell in his own clumsy way that he was trying to flirt with me. There was no place to be alone with all those people and friends around, so when he asked me to go on a ride with him I knew that's what he had in mind. Standing in line together I was in la-la land, not noticing what ride we were waiting for until it was our turn to go. Suddenly, I found myself staring at seats that belonged to the most scary-looking roller coaster I'd ever seen. I looked at him and said, 'There's no way in "h" I'm getting on that thing!' He put his arm around me, squeezed me gently and said, 'Don't worry, scaredy-cat, I'll protect you.'

"All my fears were gone as we slowly started to move. I was so mushy in love, or lust or whatever, with this guy that we could have been sitting on the top of a live volcano and I wouldn't have cared. While we were being pulled to the top, I kept trying to sneak a look at him without trying to be too obvious. A couple of times out of the corner of my eye I could see him turn toward me and start to say something, but he would lose his nerve at the last moment and turn back. His shyness only got me going even more; I really wanted him badly! At that time, I was still a virgin. But I swear to you…if I was ever going to make love to anyone in my life…it had to be him! It's amazing what lust can do to you.

"Here we were, three hundred feet in the air in this little car, and all I could do was think of him…that is, until I was abruptly jolted back to reality as the cars suddenly jerked. We hadn't quite reached the top, yet the jerk was really strong. As we continued to climb I asked him if something was wrong with the ride. He reassured me it was nothing more than the chain taking up slack. Just then we jerked again; this time it was strong enough for us to grab on to keep from sliding all over the place. My left hand held on to the side of the car, while my right reached for the bar in front of me. Kevin put one hand on the seat (between us) and the other onto the same bar. Even though we were now holding on, when the car jerked again I was tossed around a little anyway, sliding forward in my seat. The ride began to smooth out again, except for a few little bumps. It was during one of those little bumps that I suddenly realized where his hand had come to rest!

"In all the confusion when he put his hand down on the seat to catch himself it didn't land between us…instead, it landed between my legs! And what made matters worse was that during the last big tug when I slid forward, his hand slipped past my baggy shorts, and my bare crotch came to rest right on the back of his hand!

"Suddenly I froze...however, my mind was going 220 miles per hour; was this really happening? I didn't know what to think. Should I be embarrassed, should I be excited? Hell, the only thing I did know was I was scared to death. You want to talk about butterflies...anyway, I didn't know what to do. As we continued to climb, the motion caused me to rub gently back and forth on the back of his arm. I wondered if he knew what was going on? Could he have done this on purpose? Well, any thoughts that it might have been done with intention were soon swept away when he turned to me and started talking casually about God knows what. Believe me, by then I wasn't hearing anything anyway. All at once, right in the middle of some senseless sentence, he suddenly stopped talking. Out of the corner of my eye I saw him turn straight ahead and stiffen up. I guess he finally realized just where his hand was! After more than a few awkward moments had passed I mustered up enough courage to turn and look at him. We were obviously connected that day, no pun intended, because at the same time he turned to look at me. When we looked at each other I saw more fright and confusion in his eyes than there probably was in mine. I could tell he wanted to say something. I did, too, but nothing was coming out. The feel of his hand against me and the way he looked was too much for me to take. I wanted to let him know I wasn't angry and that it was all right, but all I could do was smile. I guess that was enough, for I saw relief come over his face and a weak smile come to his lips. It was like being in a trance as we moved closer...then just as our lips touched, we went over the top."

SMELL

Are there any scents that you find particularly arousing?

You may find that there are several. I have found that women's sense of smell is much more acute than men's. Women also are more capable of attaching significance to odors and are more acutely attuned to the connection that odors have with their emotions. Men seldom associate a particular perfume with a particular woman, whereas women can easily associate a variety of scents with particular places, people, or events.

Now, search your memory for any smells that make you feel romantic or erotic. For example, one woman said that every time she smelled seawater, she remembered a certain sexy experience she had with a lover on a foggy day at the beach. Another woman became aroused when she was exposed to stale cigarette smoke and heavy coffee. This stems from an experience she had in a tiny coffeehouse when she met an exciting person. One woman recalled catching a whiff of a stranger's cologne on a busy city street. It immediately whisked her back in time to her first serious love interest—who always wore Polo by Ralph Lauren aftershave:

"I'd been in love with this incredible man, and I always liked the way he smelled. But I never gave it much thought. I didn't realize the effect it could have on me until that day when the scent took me by surprise. My mind was flashing back and spinning so fast I forgot to cross the street when the light changed. Now, my nose is always on the alert."

You may find that several scents affect you in a sensual way. Remember that scents that affect you can come from the most unlikely sources, from foods to pine trees to colognes to kitchen cleansers. So keep your mind open. For every scent you list, write an explanation and a brief story about why you find it arousing.

1.

2.

3.

Here are some sample answers:

1. **Vanilla:** "I was with this very handsome man at a quaint little restaurant. It was kind of French nouveau, and we were sitting at a corner table by a window that overlooked the street. It was getting late and the place was beginning to thin out. We had finished a great meal, and he ordered us both an almond-vanilla milk, which is steamed milk, fragrant with almond and vanilla extract.

   "The milk was really hot, and the glass was very full, so when he went to grab it he pulled his hand back quickly, accidentally spilling some of the milk onto the table. I reached over to help wipe it up. He looked so cute, just like a little boy who made a big mess at the kitchen table and was sitting there waiting for his mother to scold him. Well, being the flirt that I am, while helping wipe up the spill, I grabbed him by his tie and pulled his head slowly across the table. But instead of scolding him, I gave him a killer of a kiss! The vanilla and almond scent was overpowering. That was the sweetest, best smelling kiss I ever had. Now, anytime I smell vanilla or almond extract, I relive that moment and that kiss."
2. **Cigarette Smoke:** "I know it's not politically correct, but my first love smoked like a chimney, and when we made out in his car, it just reeked. To this day, though I don't smoke and know it's not good for you, the smell of cigarettes reminds me of my young days of making out."
3. **The Smell of Pine:** "We made out in the woods, in a pine forest. The smell was overpowering. Even the odor of Pine-Sol now makes me feel sexy."

TASTE

Are there any tastes that remind you of something romantic or erotic?

Even though the sense of taste is just as sensitive as the others, its stimulation is more often directional and elicits the fewest number of sensual responses. Nonetheless, many people find that particular tastes can bring back sharp memories.

Take some time with this one, and if you happen to find a flavor or taste that reminds you of an arousing experience, write it down. Also remember to write a detailed explanation of it.

1. ______________________________

____

____

____

____

____

2. ______________________________

3. ______________________________

Here are some sample answers:

1. **Gum:** "He always carried some gum in his pocket, and his breath always smelled sweet. I remember the first time he kissed me. We were walking on Oak Street downtown after being out on the town, drinking and dancing. I was a little drunk and a little loud. I told him I was going to show him how to cross the street 'city style.' I started to jaywalk across without looking for traffic and didn't notice a cab coming straight at me. Suddenly I felt a strong hand on my shoulder, and he pulled me off the street just in time. I lost my balance and held on to him. When I finally lifted my head to say I was sorry for being such a jerk, he kissed me. He was a great kisser, and even though I was more than a little looped, I remember his mouth tasted of Clorets. It left quite an impression on me. I always have a pack of Clorets in my purse."
2. **Cognac:** "It had been a great date. We were at a wonderful restaurant. The food had been excellent, and they played soft music. We had candles on the table, and the place was decorated in English Tudor. It was very expensive and elegant. Bill ordered me a glass of Louis XIII cognac. The whole evening was perfect. I had never had cognac before, and it was great. It was warm in my mouth, and the taste lingered a long time. Now whenever I'm out to dinner and I want to really get 'in the mood' I have a glass of Louie. That's it. I'm really ready for anything."
3. **Salt:** "It was a blistering hot day, and we were making out in the shade of a willow tree. Every kiss was salty. Our bodies glistened with sweat, and when the occasional cool breeze came by, it felt wonderful. I began kissing his neck and chest, and again,

the salty taste just drove me nuts. It excited him, too, because we made love like never before. Sometimes I'll put a few salt grains in my hand and lick them up…mmm…the memories."

TOUCH

Does the feel of anything in particular against your body turn you on? Does touching anything in particular evoke romantic feelings?

Remember when answering this question that your responses can come from anything you touch and anything that touches you. Take your time and give a detailed explanation of your responses.

1. ____________________

2. ____________________

3. ____________________

Here are some sample answers:

1. **Whiskers:** "I love the rough, sandpapery feel of a man's chin when he needs a shave. I just want to rub my face and body against him."
2. **Silk:** "The feel of it against my bare skin. When I wear a silk blouse without a bra, the cool sliding of the material against my nipples keeps me excited all day. I fantasize about walking into a business meeting in a large boardroom. I'm dressed very chic: a long business suit with the jacket open, over a beige silk blouse with no bra on underneath. And around my neck is draped a long single gold chain. They can definitely tell that I am braless. I get everyone's attention, and nobody gets anything worthwhile done."
3. **Hair:** "I wear my hair long, and in the summer especially I like the feel of it when I put my hair up. I pull it tight. I love that tugging feeling at the back of my neck and the coolness. It feels like I'm naked and everyone else is dressed. It makes me feel naughty and excited at the same time. And I go into ecstasy when the man I'm with slowly takes the pins out and lets my hair down."
4. **Hair:** "I love it when my hairdresser brushes my hair, shampoos it, combs it, runs it through his fingers."
5. **Hair:** "I once had a lover who had long, thick hair. I had taken off my shirt and was lying on the floor. He was giving me a back rub. All of a sudden, I felt the most incredible feeling across my back. He was rubbing his hair over me. It was the most unbelievable feeling. I was out of the rest of my clothes in two seconds, and he touched me with his hair on every part of my body. It felt like I'd died and gone to heaven. Now I even get excited sometimes when I feel my own hair on my shoulders."
6. **Tight Underwear:** "I love the way it feels when I pull a pair of panties high up on my waist; I love that snugness between my legs. At times when I do that I feel sexy all day long, even if I'm at work."
7. **Popsicles:** "I like the way a Popsicle feels. I enjoy the way the cold feels on my lips and how it starts to melt and get sloppy. Ice itself doesn't do it for me, it has to be a Popsicle. I get a nasty, wicked feeling when I eat one. If they weren't so fattening, I'd eat a dozen of them every day."
8. **Kneading Bread:** "When I knead bread, it feels like I'm kneading a man's...well, you know! I make fantastic breads because I put so much energy into kneading."

SOUND

Are there any sounds that elicit your sensual thoughts or feelings? Are there any songs or music that do the same? What puts you "in the mood for love"?

Hearing is one of the strongest senses. Sounds have been shown to initiate our mental imaging process and have been shown to possess a more intense effect than any other non-human stimulation. Sounds such as music have a special link with our emotions (that link is so special that we will deal with sound and music more thoroughly in Chapter Nine). In a person's life, certain songs can be associated with nearly every emotion and human condition. Memories of school, work, vacations, sorrow, hate, and love can be elicited by a particular sound or music.

Because sounds and music can elicit such a wide variety of responses, it is important to narrow our selection to those sounds and music that will bring out the particular emotion we are looking for—sensual!

1. ____

2. ____

3. ____

____

____

____

____

____

____

____

____

Here are some sample answers:

1. **(Song) "A Girl Like You:"** "I was going out with this guy I was crazy about. We had gone on a trip to California and just about every song I hear from that time reminds me of it. But there is one in particular. We went to this new dance club in Palm Springs. We had been there a while, just sitting at a table watching other people dance. We hadn't danced even once yet when this slow song began to play by Foreigner, "A Girl Like You." It was then he looked at me in the cutest way and asked me if I would dance with him. We did. And as we were moving it felt like we were one person. It really did! I can still picture the way he looked at me and smiled. Now when I hear that song, or any song by that group, I'm history. I'll start remembering everything. Even though the first thing I think about when I hear it isn't some hot and heavy sex scene, it really turns me on when I think about it."
2. **(Song) "Lady in Red:"** "I was on my second date with Rob, and we went to this cozy little cafe where they had a small dance floor. As it happened, I was wearing a new red dress, and I knew it looked great on me. Rob seemed not to notice it, until "Lady in Red" came on. We danced to it, and he kept holding me tighter and tighter. Whenever I hear that song, I remember how sexy and desirable I felt that night."
3. **Madonna:** "We were in bed making love for the first time. I had put a Madonna tape in right before things started getting good. Then once they started to get hot and heavy I didn't want to break the mood by getting up to change the tape, so it played over and over. But the best part was when things started to calm down and we started to become aware of our surroundings again. It was then we heard Madonna singing "Like a Virgin." We tried to sing along with her but it just made us laugh all the harder. Anyway, whenever I hear one of her songs, it sure puts me in a good mood!"

Sounds that can elicit a romantic response are not confined to music. When you are searching your memory, think about everyday sounds that might do the job. For example, voices, bells, thunder, trains, birds, and so forth. Keep an open mind—and an open ear—when you review your experiences.

4. **Crickets:** "We were out camping. There was a little fire going, we had just eaten, and we started slowly making love. The sky was black, the stars were huge…but most of all, the crickets were going crazy. It was like nature was serenading us and trying to make everything just perfect. To this day, I love the sound of crickets."
5. **Voices and Thunder:** "I never really liked thunder. I had a dog who was deathly afraid of it. I even had to give him Valium to knock him out each time there was a thunderstorm. Well, I was out on a date with a really good-looking man who had a great voice, soft and deep. It was spring, and after dinner we went outside and started walking when it began to storm. We ran under a large green awning right beside this huge tree to wait it out. It started to get very windy and started to thunder and lightning heavily. I got a little frightened and reached up under his suit coat and put my arms around his waist to hold on to him. I guess I was shaking or something, because he could tell I was frightened. He put his arms around me and said in a calming low voice: "Don't worry, everything will be all right." The way he sounded, so calm and sure. The way he felt, so solid and strong. And the way he smelled, fresh, made me feel safer than I ever felt before. We finally made our way to my place and made some thunder and lightning of our own. I've never been afraid of thunder since. Now whenever I hear it I think of that night. And I'm a sucker for a deep voice. Even at work, I noticed I've developed an affinity for people who have a nice voice. They can always get my attention."

After you have completed this questionnaire, go back over your answers and select one or two that you find most arousing. As you continue with your lessons you will use several of your answers, but for now I want you to narrow your selection to just a couple. From these you are to pick just one response—the one that you find most arousing. You will draw upon this selection in the exercises that follow. After you feel completely at ease with your selection, go on to Chapter Five. However, if you are unsure that you have completed the questionnaire properly, go over the instructions at the beginning of this chapter and try again before proceeding. If you are unsure that the response that you have chosen is suitable, remember that the most important criterion in choosing your response is: "Do you find it arousing?" At this point nothing else is important. If you are still not satisfied, read Chapters Seven and Eight on fantasy and vision before continuing with the next chapter. Again, remember that you're not trying to write great literature, although you may be surprised at how literary you get. Your aim is to create or re-create a vivid erotic image.

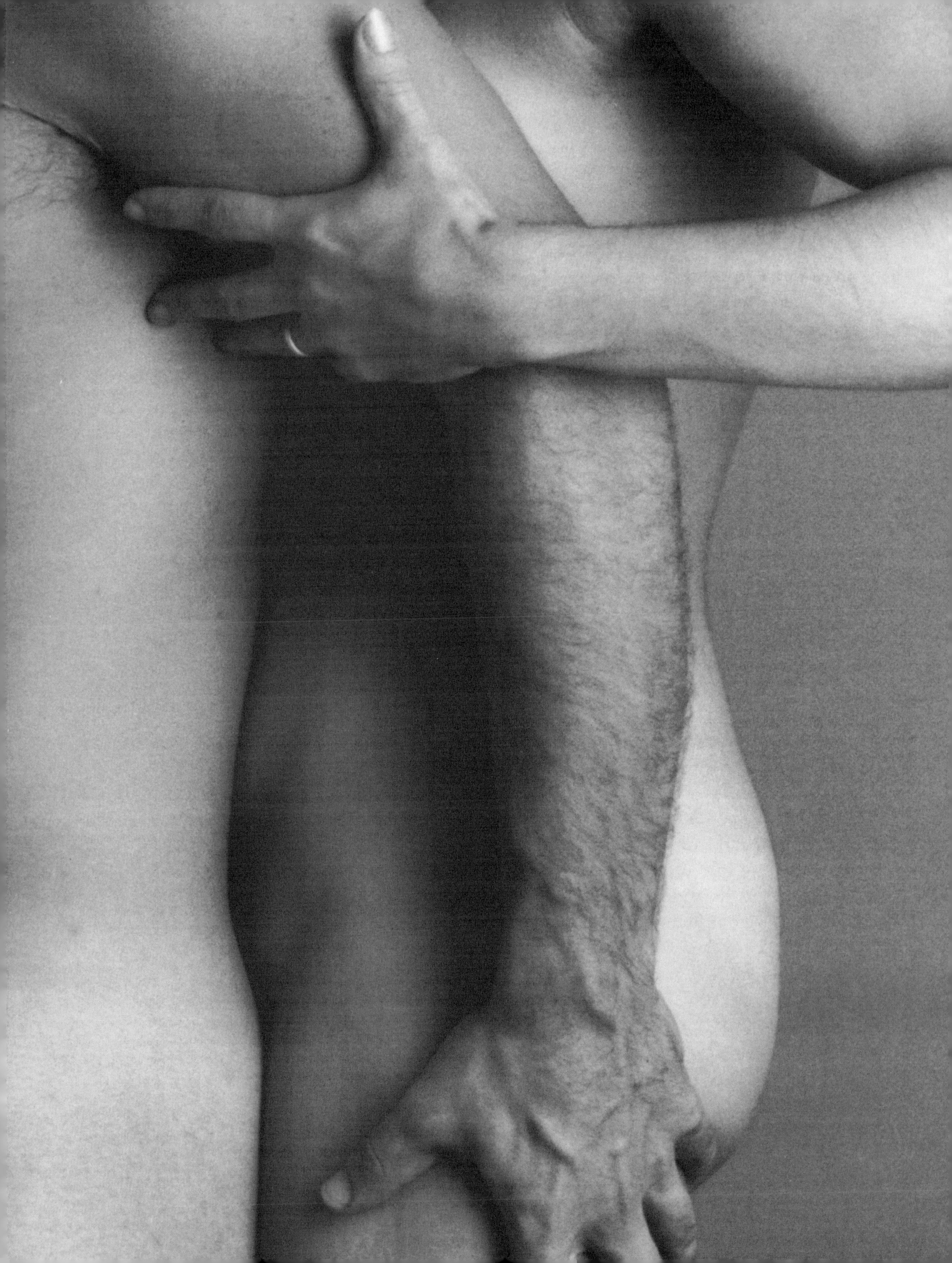

5

Chapter Five

Person to Person

Most self-help books leave you pretty much on your own. Often their instructions are too complicated or too vague to be of any real help. With such books, if you are unclear about something and need to ask a question, you have nowhere to turn. To avoid this, I have tried to answer any questions that you might ask. These answers will be comprehensive and will lessen the possibility that you will become frustrated with your therapy and give up.

While interviewing patients, I have noticed that several questions routinely surface. I have learned that the most effective method of answering those questions is to give examples of how other patients have responded in similar situations. In this way, patients get a better understanding of what I want them to do.

At this point, I would like you to read an interview with a real patient. I am sure you will find it helpful in answering many questions that might arise while working through your Solid Therapy.

My interview took place with a woman named Julie. After having a preliminary discussion and going through the questionnaire in Chapter Four, we began.

TALKING WITH JULIE

Doctor: "Can you think of anything that makes you feel sexually excited?"

Julie: "What do you mean?"

Doctor: "Is there some event, real-life experience, or fantasy, that can cause you to feel some excitement?"

Julie: "Well, yes. I guess there is, but I can't just sit and think of something and get myself excited."

Doctor: "What do you mean?"

Julie: "You know, we've talked about it before. I need some time to relax. I need some time to unwind and clear my head before I can get in the mood."

Doctor: "OK, let's say ideally you are at home or the place where you feel the most comfortable. You have had all the time you needed to get rid of things that bothered you during the day. Let me ask you again…provided the environment is right, is there anything you can think of that will cause you to get excited?"

Julie: "Yeah, sure!"

Doctor: "Can you be more specific? Is it something that you've thought about more than once?"

Julie: "Yes."

Doctor: "Is this a particular real-life experience or a fantasy?"

Julie: "An event. It's something that happened to me a while ago."

Doctor: "And it's something that you have thought about more than once or twice?"

Julie: "I do have a particular event that causes me to get excited when I think about it…but everything else has to be all right first, you know."

Doctor: "So you have at least one recurrent theme that you can think about, provided your environment is relaxed, that will cause you to get excited?"

Julie: "Yes, it's usually the same thing. Sometimes I think about it when I'm making love, too. And sometimes it's a little different."

Doctor: "How do you mean?"

Julie: "Sometimes the story varies a little."

Doctor: "Is it a completely different one?"

Julie: "No. It's basically the same one, but sometimes little things are different. Like a different time of day or a different house."

Doctor: "OK, so we know that there is at least one event that gets you excited when you think about it. Let me ask you if there are any other events or things that are able to do the same. Or is there only one?"

Julie: "Oh, no, there are a couple more things that I can think about that can get me excited. Since the questionnaire, I've been thinking about it. I know there are a couple of others. But the one we've been talking about is the one that I think about most often and gets to me the most."

Doctor: "OK, now let's get a little more specific. I would like for you to tell me what it is that you think about that can get you excited."

Julie: "All of them?"

Doctor: "No. Let's start with the one that gets you most excited. The one that you said comes to mind more often than the others."

Julie: "Oh, that. OK, well, there is this guy and myself in this room on a big couch. We are kissing and things started to get a little carried away, then it gets really hot."

Doctor: "The room you mentioned, is it important to the story as well or will any room do?"

Julie: "Oh, yeah, it's important. It's his den. It was just what you would imagine a den should be like. An Old English-style den, with books all over the walls, a beautiful old desk, and a huge couch."

Doctor: "What I would like you to try to do is to tell me what picture comes to mind when you first start thinking about it."

Julie: "Well, I guess we're on the couch kissing and..."

Doctor: "Stop! Let me ask you in another way. When you are by yourself or making love or whatever, and you begin to think about this particular experience, let's say you have a Polaroid camera and are able to take a picture of the very first thought that actually comes to your mind. This is what I would like for you to describe to me."

Julie: "I don't know if I can. I really haven't thought about it like that."

Doctor: "Well, when you start to think about anything, there is an initial image that comes to your mind. But many times we never focus our attention on it because it's usually not important that we do. Let's go on. Can you tell me how the two of you are dressed?"

Julie: "Well..."

Doctor: "Are the two of you dressed?"

Julie: "Kind of."

Doctor: "Let's try something else that might help. Are the two of you lying on the couch, just sitting, or..."

Julie: "We're sitting on the couch."

Doctor: "Is it an average couch?"

Julie: "Oh, no. It was neat. It was a beautiful dark reddish leather one, burgundy! It had a big, heavy, padded, rounded back and arms with spaced buttons all through it, except the cushions; they were heavy and smooth."

Doctor: "That was great! You see, you can do it. Your description of the couch was terrific. However, I think you could use a little time to think about it. I know this is new to you, so I want you to take some time and study that imaginary picture. When we meet again I want you to be able to describe it to me in detail, as if you are describing it right from a photograph. And remember, the picture you are taking is of the very first thought that comes to mind when you begin thinking about it."

Our next meeting the following week:

Julie: "I've been thinking about it. Sometimes the story jumps and it doesn't always go in the same sequence, and at times I think about things that happened toward the end of the story, but there is one thing that usually comes to mind first when I start thinking about it."

Doctor: "Can you tell me what that is and describe it like you are describing a picture of it?"

Julie: "Sure, I'll try. We're at his home; it's about 7:30 P.M., in his den. The only light that was on was a green shaded lamp on his desk. The walls were covered with shelves, books, and pictures. Some of the shelves had different knickknacks."

Doctor: "What kind of knickknacks?"

Julie: "There was a beautiful crystal clock that chimed every fifteen minutes. A small easel with a picture of him and some friends on vacation. Several black, deerlike figurines that he bought while on another trip. There were pictures on the walls staggered in between the books and shelves. Some of the pictures didn't seem to fit in with the decor, but those stood out and caught my eye. I'm sure that's why I noticed them first, because they were different. He had sketches of parrots and pictures of old European houses. One lithograph was of Beethoven's home. The ones that stood out were by Patrick Nagel. I told you they made an impression on me. His desk was old and made of dark rosewood. Another small easel was on it with a picture of his family. There were also a couple of books open, along with several books between stone horse-head bookends. One side of the room had full-length terrace doors. They were open."

Doctor: "Do you remember what the weather was like?"

Julie: "That was one of the best parts. It was still light out but very dark because it was about to storm. You could hear thunder and see lightning far off. And every so often the wind would blow like crazy."

Doctor: "And where were you?"

Julie: "Like I said before, we were on his leather couch. I was sitting in the corner of it with my left arm on the armrest. He had given me a glass of Bailey's. It was the first time I tried it. He had a small glass, too."

Doctor: "How were you dressed?"

Julie: "He had taken off his jacket and had on a white shirt with the sleeves rolled up. His tie was loosened around his neck. He had on great suspenders. A small black watch on his left wrist stood out. Boy, did he ever look sexy! He was sitting real close to me with one knee bent up on the couch, touching my thigh."

Doctor: "How were you dressed?"

Julie: "Oh! I had on an Anne Klein gray linen evening suit, buttoning low on the waist. Under it I had on a silk off-white blouse, with a gold and pearl necklace. I had unbuttoned the top of my blouse and tucked my necklace inside. I pulled my lapels open and loosened up my jacket so I would look a little more sexy. I made sure you could see the top of my lace bra. It was white."

Doctor: "You're doing great! Is there anything else?"

Julie: "Oh, yeah, like I said, he was sitting next to me with his knee touching my right thigh, and his left hand was touching my hair and neck. Well, things started to get good.

Between the sounds of the storm, the wind, and him, it was something else! We did some unbelievable things on that couch."

Julie continued with her story, adding more details to her picture. She also described other parts of her experience that she thought of often and found arousing.

Now let me ask *you* a question: Provided that you are in a place that allows you to feel comfortable, is there one particular experience or scenario that elicits erotic feelings when you think about it? The experience or scenario can come from a past event, from a favorite fantasy, or from a combination of both. What you find arousing isn't important just yet, nor is when and where you think about your particular experience. Also, it makes no difference whether you've thought about it when alone, when making love, or when at the Laundromat during the middle of the day. What is important is, first, that it be a recurrent thought, and, second, that it elicit sensual or erotic feelings. Write down your answer in the spaces that follow. If you can think of more than one answer, briefly write down those as well, but the first one should be the experience or scenario that recurs most often and that arouses you the most. Then list the remainder of them, if any. More space is available in the Workbook Section that begins on page 159.

Before you write down your responses, be sure you have completed the questionnaire in Chapter Four and read the following initial responses from Julie.

Can you think of anything that has the ability to get you aroused?

1. **House in Skokie:** Stan and I on his large leather couch (kissing) in his den on a stormy afternoon-evening.
2. **South Florida:** Walking on the beach (early morning). Look for shells on Marco Island. Then making love in the open.

Now write down your answers.

1. ______________________________

____

____

____

____

____

2. ______________________________

____

____

3.

SNAPSHOT RECOLLECTION

Now go over your responses and think about the one that you have singled out as most arousing. Describe the first thought that comes to your mind when you think about it, as if you are looking at a snapshot. That snapshot should be the first image that comes to your mind. In a moment I will ask you to write down your recollection of that snapshot image in the spaces that follow, including as much detail as you can. I do not want you to write down a continuation of the story. What is important here is to confine yourself to describing (on paper) the initial image.

Using the following instructions, here is how Julie completed her snapshot recollection:

1. **Describe the picture that first comes to your mind.**
2. **Describe it as if you were describing a snapshot of the first thought that jumps into your mind whenever you think of the event.**
3. **Fill in with as much detail as you can.**

> Cloudy, stormy June late afternoon—sitting in his den lit only by his desk lamp. The walls were lined with bookshelves and pictures. The shelves were full of books, knick-knacks, and little pictures. A large set of French doors were slightly open and we could see the lightning and hear the thunder.

Many people have noticed that different snapshot scenes come to mind about the same event. In our example, Julie vividly remembered several scenes from this particular adventure. However, even though Julie could clearly visualize more than one arousing scene, she did not mix up her descriptions of them. She kept them separate. When you are describing a particular "snapshot," do not combine it with another that you find arousing. Confine your description to one picture at a time, not a continuous depiction of your experience.

This is a very important step, so take all the time you need and be thorough. Don't worry if you take quite a while to complete your material. As we've seen with Julie, as well as with many other women, it's not easy at first. Although the picture may be something that you often think about, bringing it to a conscious level and describing it in detail may be difficult.

If you have trouble expressing your snapshot, go over the interview with Julie again and ask yourself questions similar to those that were asked of her. Or go through Chapter Six, which includes detailed descriptions of other women's snapshots.

If you still are not sure how to do it, it may help if you page through a few books or magazines and find a picture that resembles your particular snapshot. I call this a *Visual Subsidy*, which is described in greater detail in Chapter Eight. Keep that book or magazine picture next to you while you are writing down the description of your snapshot. Use the picture to bring to your attention the differences as well as the similarities between the two. This method helps you to focus your thoughts and makes it easier for you to visualize the sensual ideas that you are trying to describe.

Now it's your turn, Follow, as Julie did, these instructions in writing down your snapshot recollection:

1. **Describe the picture that first comes to your mind.**
2. **Describe it as if you were describing a snapshot of the first thought that jumps into your mind whenever you think of the event.**
3. **Fill in with as much detail as you can.**

Snapshot Recollection:

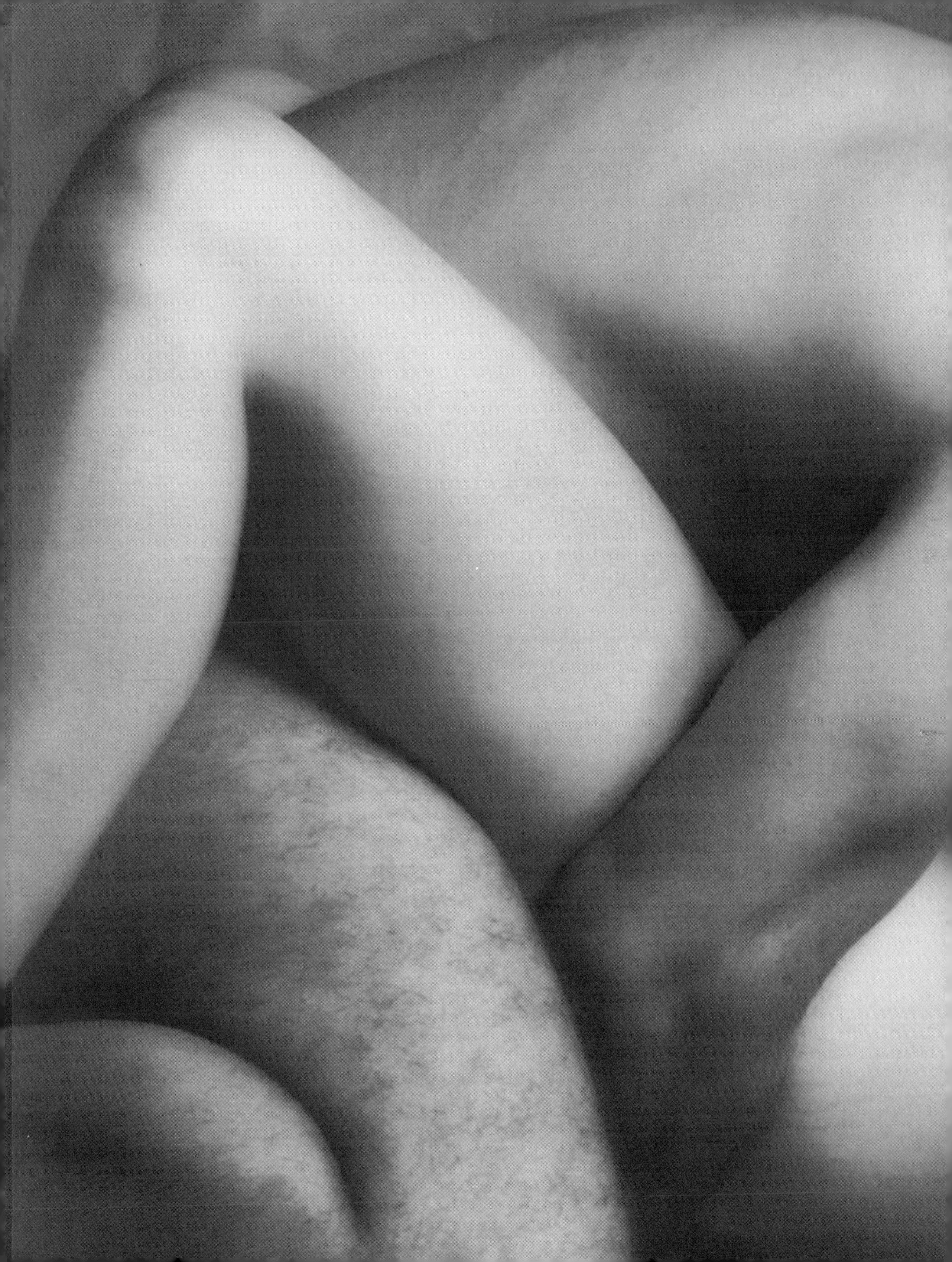

6

Chapter Six

Case Study

Often the responses that women give to the questions in Chapter Five are not "camera ready," that is, not in a clear, focused format before the women attempt the exercises. I want to reemphasize that the description that you wrote down in Chapter Five should be that of a snapshot—a single picture of the first thought that comes to your mind when you begin to remember the arousing event, not a continuation of the event. If your written response is not a clear description of a snapshot, rewrite it before you proceed.

CASE STUDY OF CONNIE

So that you can be certain that you properly completed the exercises in Chapter Five, we will go through a sample case study in detail. Following is the case study of a patient named Connie. First is her initial response when asked, as Julie was, to select the recollection that she found most arousing.

Connie's answer: "Flowers and gardens."

Connie's initial response: "I was in my garden, in the backyard of my house, clipping leaves around some peonies. It was really hot, and I was wearing a small print tank top and pale printed shorts, sandals, and garden gloves. My boyfriend came home and saw me messing around in the garden again and made some comment on how he wished I paid as much attention to him as I did my flowers. I felt like being a little bitchy, and because I was on my knees already, I simply bent over and wiggled my butt in the air and made some stupid comment like, 'How would you like to prune this flower, big boy?'

"Before I could look around to check his reaction he came right up behind me. He grabbed my butt with one hand and slipped his other right onto my chest. It really startled me because I didn't think he was that close! Well, I jumped in reaction to his scaring me and twisted around quickly. When I did, his hand got trapped in my shorts, and the momentum caught him off balance, taking him down to his knees, causing his clean clothes to get full of dirt. I told him I was sorry but that it was his fault for scaring me. And that I wasn't in the mood to fool around anyway because it was too hot and I felt all sweaty and grubby. Well, as he was getting up he seemed more than just a little irritated, and as he was turning away I could faintly hear him say something about me always being the wrong kind of hot and walked back into the house to clean up, at least so I thought.

"I had gone back to my clipping and was still on my knees when all at once I felt a blast of cold water hitting me. I turned to see that he had put the sprinkler on me and was taking his shirt off as he ran up behind me again to put his arms around me, preventing me from getting away from the water. He said maybe this would cool me off. Before I could say anything, we were getting all wet and muddy, and he kissed me! Well, after a few seconds of that, mixed in with the feel of his warm, soft skin and what his hands started to do to me, I didn't care if I was hot and sweaty or wet and muddy. I felt kind of animal-like. We made love there, ruining our clothes and part of the garden, but I didn't care. I love the feel of rain on me now.

"I remember trying to escape from the sprinkler drops by attempting to hide under his body like an umbrella. I couldn't get all the way under him, and some of the drops would hit my arms and legs. I can remember feeling the peonies I had picked earlier underneath me. I could feel their soft petals touch the small of my back when we moved back and forth. I remember while I was lying under him hiding from the sprinkler, that I turned my head slightly to one side and while I felt his body covering mine, I was watching how the water from the sprinkler was hitting the nearby fence, then running down and how the moisture was soaking into the wood in a funny pattern around three large knots. Then after a little time had passed I pushed him over and rolled on top of him, letting the water rinse me off and cool me down."

As you can see, Connie told a story of the entire event as she remembered it. After reviewing her initial response, Connie was told to write a second draft of her description of the event, following as closely as possible these instructions:

1. **Describe the picture of what first comes to your mind when you begin to remember the event.**
2. **Describe this first thought as if you were describing a "snapshot" of that first image that jumps into your mind whenever you think of the event.**
3. **Take your time when describing your snapshot and provide as much detail as possible. The reasons will become obvious as we proceed. At this point I just want to remind you that details are very important.**

Connie continued and made a second draft as instructed:

"The picture in my mind is that of a sunny day; it had a very hot, late-summery feeling. My back yard and garden are very picturesque. It's bordered on one side by the back of my house; the house's facade is made up of cream-colored painted bricks, with many dark brown-framed shuttered windows. There are wide patches of deep green ivy spreading over sections of the wall. Light and dark pink peonies line part of the wall under a large green and white curtained window that belongs to my sun room. A cream-painted wooden patio door opens onto the patio. The patio floor itself is made with bricks arranged in a vibrant pattern. Due to their age, the bricks had settled, developing small spaces between each one, just wide enough to let tiny blades of grass grow between them. On the patio there are several pieces of white wicker patio furniture, a couple of chairs with light-colored, floral-printed cushions, and a matching table and magazine rack. Not far away is a black grill with a metal holder attached that keeps all the barbecue paraphernalia neatly organized. Next to the back door is a green, rolled-up garden hose hanging low on the side of the house. Except for an area bordering the garden itself, which is lined by a high unpainted wooden fence, evergreens and tall bushes surround the remainder of the house and garden. The yard looks like a dark green, thick carpet, neatly manicured and edged.

"A narrow curved cement walk splits the yard into two large sections, with two rather substantial, noble-looking oak trees placed in the middle of each section. There is one spot on the wooden fence lining the garden that has three rather large, distinctive-looking knots, one stacked right above the other just slightly touching each other. The garden itself has a section abutting the patio with a perennial border of campanula, sedum, phlox, lady's mantle, and Jacob's ladder. Another section has stately junipers, tall grasses, and many varieties of iris. In my picture I am there, on my hands and knees in my lightly printed shorts and top, with off-white sandals and white floral-printed work gloves. On my left side there are light pink peonies with broken stems that I had picked earlier. Alongside of that is my toolbox, filled with my garden tools and assorted garden goodies."

Can you see how Connie's second description of her thoughts was much better? She was giving a direct physical description of the snapshot rather than telling the story behind the snapshot. Her description of events can now be better used for her Solid Therapy lessons. You can create your own format or use hers as a guide. But keep in mind that it is important to write down all your thoughts in a similar fashion. That is, take all of your unorganized, often vague feelings about that one arousing memory or fantasy and force yourself to recount as many details as possible, then write them down into an organized, concrete representation.

Take some time and write down your initial recollection of a single arousing memory or fantasy. More space is available in the Workbook Section that begins on page 159.

Snapshot Recollection Part 1

Again, it is important that you carry out this initial step and follow this outline as closely as possible because it will help you to bring vague, unusable feelings into hard focus and into a concise, usable format from which you can obtain the maximum benefit.

Now we will begin to make you feel more comfortable and accustomed to thinking about sex. Are you ready? You will be attempting to undo years of well-learned, inhibited attitudes and behaviors, so be patient. We first need to get you to form mental images about sex. I have found that many women, without the proper circumstances and stimulation, go for days without having sexual thoughts.

Moreover, nearly 97 percent of women whom I questioned expressed a need for some time to erase the cares of the day before they felt comfortable enough to think about sex. This time buffer could be accomplished by taking a leisurely bubble bath, drinking a cocktail, reading a magazine, listening to music, and so forth. Switching from the role of mother, housekeeper, career woman, or caretaker to the role of *femme fatale* took a complete mental "change of scenery." The type of activity that was performed during the time wasn't important. What was important was that whatever these women did helped clear their minds, allowing them to open the doors to their libidos.

You have to *learn* to think easily and naturally about sex whenever and wherever you please, even at those times and in those places that may seem strange or unnatural for you. Think about it: Most people's mornings include showering, shaving, brushing their teeth, and so forth. But if, for whatever reason, they find themselves taking a shower in the evening, they might feel it a little strange or unnatural. Or, many people consider eggs to be strictly breakfast food and would never think of eating them at night. Yet there are millions of people who love to eat eggs for dinner. It's just a matter of what you are accustomed to. Habits help determine your prejudices and behaviors toward everything in life. And that extends to sexual thoughts.

We are going to start slowly by concentrating in a very structured way and then build upon that. The time allotted to these exercises may seem excessive. I have purposely allotted more time than is necessary for a great number of women. If you can proceed from one exercise to the next in less time, please do so. These time guidelines are the maximum requirements.

If you still have difficulty selecting and describing an arousing event of your own, read Chapters Four and Eight before continuing.

First, I want you to read the description of your snapshot that you just wrote. Next, pick out four items from your snapshot that are most prominent in your mind. These will become tools that we call Focal Items.

Now write down your Focal Items.

Focal Items:

1. ______________________________

2. ______________________________

3. ______________________________

4. ______________________________

You will probably notice, as Connie did, that more than one item in your snapshot will stand out to you. Connie had found that two items stood out: the knots in the fence and the pink peonies by her side. Don't fret over choosing one item over others because eventually you will use all of them. For now, however, narrow your choices to one Focal Item. Connie singled out the "pink peonies with broken stems."

Now write a second, more detailed recollection of your snapshot. Try to make yourself aware of details that you may have left out of your initial mental reconstruction and write those down after your second recollection. Use the space provided. Take your time.

Snapshot Recollection Part 2

____

____

____

____

____

____

____

____

Items forgotten or not included during your first recollection:

1.

2.

3.

New items remembered during your first recollection:

1.

2. ____

____

____

____

____

____

3. ____

____

____

____

____

____

At this point, put all of this material away and forget about it for a while. Eat a sandwich. Pay some bills. Go on. Shoo! Even if you are eager to proceed with your therapy, I want you to take a respite for at least an hour before continuing…

…OK. Now that you are refreshed (or possibly just stuffed and broke), let's continue. Without looking at any of your material, turn your attention to the Focal Item that you selected. After you have visualized it, begin to rebuild that snapshot as you did before. Do not look at any of your written material yet. Try to recollect all that you can with as much detail as you can. When you have done that, turn to your second written recollection and review it, just as before. Again, briefly write down all the things that you had not included and the things that you had forgotten.

Items forgotten or not included during your second recollection:

1. ____

____

____

____

____

____

2.

3.

New items remembered during your second recollection:

1.

2.

3.

Now we are going to ease you into getting accustomed to working with a schedule, starting off slowly until you feel comfortable with it. Just as some medicines must be taken three times a day for maximum effectiveness, so, too, these lessons need to be carried out at different times of the day over a period of days to help you learn a natural behavior. We will start you off in the morning, although you *may* start in the afternoon or evening.

A few simple definitions might help you: A *lesson* is the smallest unit of work done in your therapy, usually lasting from two to ten minutes. A *set* is a group of lessons done during the same part of the day (morning, afternoon, or evening). A *series* is the same set of lessons done over a period of days while using the same Focal Item or Visual Subsidy (more on Visual Subsidies in Chapter Eight).

Begin your first morning lesson by turning your attention to your first Focal Item without looking at any of your material. After you have visualized it in your mind, begin to rebuild your snapshot as you did before. Do not look at any of your written material yet. Try to recollect all that you can with as much detail as you can. When you have completed that, turn to your latest written snapshot recollection and review it as before. Again, briefly write down all of the things that you had not included in your mental reconstruction and the things that you had forgotten.

Repeat the exercise as many times as fifteen minutes will allow in the spaces that follow. Take your time and be thorough. With time you will be able to complete each lesson more easily and quickly. I have found that most lessons take between five and ten minutes. However, if you find that yours take longer than fifteen minutes, don't worry. That doesn't mean that you are slow or that you are doing them wrong. More likely, it simply means that you have a lot to think about. And that's good! Just spread out the time for each lesson.

FIRST LESSON SERIES

Snapshot Recollection Form

Lesson 1 (Morning)

Items forgotten or not included during your recollection:

1. ____

2.

3.

New items remembered during your recollection:

1.

2.

3.

After you have finished the morning lesson, put down your material and return to it in the afternoon. Pick any time that is convenient at first. If you are beginning your lessons in the evening, that's fine. However, it is important that you do your lessons during the prescribed parts of the day: morning, afternoon, and evening. The specific hour you choose is not important. But you will not receive the desired benefits if you do all your lessons during the same part of the day. Keep in mind that to alter old habits, sometimes you need to replace them with new ones. You need to begin to think erotic thoughts at unaccustomed times. For example, if you usually have most of your thoughts of sex in the evening, it is important that you do lessons both in the morning and the afternoon to change your behavioral pattern and to feel comfortable having sexual thoughts at those times. Now complete the afternoon lesson as you did the morning lesson:

Snapshot Recollection Form

Lesson 1 (Afternoon)

Items forgotten or not included during your recollection:

1.

2.

3.

New items remembered during your recollection:

1.

2.

3.

After you have finished your afternoon lesson, put your material away and return to it later that day. Pick a convenient time. Do the evening lesson as you did the earlier ones:

Snapshot Recollection Form
Lesson 1 (Evening)
Items forgotten or not included during your recollection:

1. ______________________________

2. ______________________________

3. ______________________________

New items remembered during your recollection:

1. ______________________________

2.

3.

If you find that you can't possibly set aside time (probably less than an hour a day) to do your lessons thoroughly, any amount of time that you can invest is better than nothing. And although you might not progress as quickly as you or I would like, you will benefit from the lessons nonetheless. Do what you can!

When doing your lesson set, give yourself a breather between lessons. In fact, after each lesson in a set, I want you to forget about it until you are ready to start the next lesson in that set. Therefore, doing something after each lesson—working, exercising, taking care of the house, or whatever—will help you get the most out of each lesson set.

After you have completed this series, again take a rest and clear your mind. Do not look at this material for at least one day but for not longer than two. Taking a break for any longer than two days at this point will set you back. You need to become accustomed to this type of thinking for a little longer.

When you return from your break, I want you to look over your description and pick a new Focal Item in your snapshot. Again, find something that stands out to you. If nothing stands out, any item will do. You will use this new Focal Item in the next series of lessons. You are to carry out each new lesson in the same manner as previously, except that you use this second Focal Item to reconstruct your snapshot.

Referring back to our sample case study, as you remember, Connie's first choice of Focal Item was that of the peonies that were lying by her side. For her second choice she picked the three knots in the wooden fence. This time when beginning to do her lessons, she would start by visualizing the three knots and from there reconstruct her snapshot.

Take a moment to review exactly how you are to execute your lessons.

Now do the second lesson series, using your second Focal Item, for just two days. Remember to do the lessons exactly as laid out and to take your time. After you have completed this second series, take another break. This time, however, limit your break to one day.

SECOND LESSON SERIES

Lesson 1
Items forgotten or not included during your recollection:

1. __________

2. __________

3. __________

New items remembered during your recollection:

1. ______________________________

2. ______________________________

3. ______________________________

Upon returning to your material, go over your snapshot recollection again and pick out your third Focal Item from your list. This will be used in your next series of lessons.

Now repeat your lesson sets as you have learned them for the next two days. For example, for her third Focal Item, Connie selected the faded red patio bricks. From that she completed a reconstruction of her picture. When you have completed the third lesson series, take a day to relax.

THIRD LESSON SERIES

Lesson 1

Items forgotten or not included during your recollection:

1.

2.

3.

New items remembered during your recollection:

1.

2.

3.

As before, after you have completed your third set of lessons and your break, begin the process again. Choose a fourth Focal Item from your snapshot description and use that for the fourth series of lessons. In our sample case study, Connie chose the green and white curtains in the porch window, from which she reconstructed her snapshot. Then, as before, repeat the lesson sets for two days and rest for one.

FOURTH LESSON SERIES

Lesson 1
Items forgotten or not included during your recollection:

1.

2.

3.

New items remembered during your recollection:

1.

2.

3. ______________________________

____

____

____

____

____

____

Here is your recommended schedule:

First lesson series: A ten-minute lesson set, made up of two to four lessons, done three times a day—morning, afternoon, and evening—for a total minimum of thirty minutes a day. Rest one day.

Second lesson series: A ten-minute lesson set, made up of two to four lessons, done three times a day—morning, afternoon, and evening—for a total minimum of thirty minutes a day. Rest one day.

Third lesson series: A ten-minute lesson set, made up of two to four lessons, done three times a day—morning, afternoon, and evening—for a total minimum of thirty minutes a day. Rest one day.

Fourth lesson series: A ten-minute lesson set, made up of two to four lessons, done three times a day—morning, afternoon, and evening—for a total minimum of thirty minutes a day. Stop.

- **Here are the forms. There is space for only two lessons for each part of the day. If you do more lessons per set, more space is available in the Workbook Section.**

Snapshot Recollection Form

Lesson 1 (Morning)

Items forgotten or not included during your recollection:

1. ______________________________

____

____

____

____

____

2.

3.

New items remembered during your recollection:

1.

2.

3.

Lesson 2 (Morning)

Items forgotten or not included during your recollection:

1.

2.

3.

New items remembered during your recollection:

1.

2.

3.

Lesson 1 (Afternoon)
Items forgotten or not included during your recollection:

1.

2.

3.

New items remembered during your recollection:

1.

2.

3. ______

Lesson 2 (Afternoon)
Items forgotten or not included during your recollection:

1. ______

2. ______

3. ______

New items remembered during your recollection:

1.

2.

3.

Lesson 1 (Evening)
Items forgotten or not included during your recollection:

1.

2.

3.

New items remembered during your recollection:

1.

2.

3.

Lesson 2 (Evening)

Items forgotten or not included during your recollection:

1.

2.

3.

New items remembered during your recollection:

1.

2.

3.

As we proceed with this next part of the therapy, we will continue to use your original snapshot. However, this time we will use it in a slightly different fashion. Go through your snapshot description and select a Focal Item that stands out to you. Then write down your description and visualize the item.

Brief Snapshot Recollection Form

Focal Item:

Description:

Now mentally reconstruct your picture as you have before. However, this time do it quickly. And don't include as much detail as you did before. I want you to have a mental image of your picture when you are finished. Remember this time not to mentally acknowledge details as you did earlier. Instead, if you have completed the first part of your therapy, you should be able to get a mental image of your picture by conceptualizing your chosen Focal Item, and then briefly visualizing the scene.

Now we are going to put some life back into your picture. After you have briefly visualized your snapshot and have a mental image of it, let's take it a frame farther. That is, think about what happened next during the event that your snapshot is based on. Think about what that snapshot leads to. In other words, so far you have reconstructed a snapshot from an event that you find arousing. Now I want you to imagine that your snapshot is the beginning frame of a motion picture: the first scene, if you will, of a movie. *Your* movie! Next you will turn on the movie, sit back, and watch what happens. Lights! Camera! Action!

Let's go back to our sample case study. For the second step in her therapy, Connie chose the Focal Item that she had used before—that of the peonies lying by her side. She began her lesson by visualizing the flowers as she remembered, then she began to reconstruct the picture mentally. As she was instructed, she took much less time than before. She could do that because she had become familiar with the process of mental reconstruction, which made it easier for her. This time, while making her mental picture, she did not have to take the time to visualize every detail. After visualizing herself kneeling in the garden on that hot day, she next remembered her boyfriend sneaking up behind and her grabbing her, putting one hand down her shorts and the other hand up her shirt. Then she remembered being startled and twisting around and knocking him to the ground. She went on to remember what they said and her thinking that he went into the house to clean up, then suddenly feeling the cold water from the sprinkler hitting her. She remembered how it felt when they were making love, how the mud was all over, and how their clothes were twisted, bunched up in a mess. She recalled what was going through her mind, having no clothes on, making love like crazy, getting all muddy in her back yard, ruining part of her garden, and all this in broad daylight.

Then she remembered how she felt not caring that she was tearing up part of her garden, how dangerous it felt to be out in the open, and how she felt nasty and wonderful at the same time for doing what she was doing. She continued with her recollection of the incident, remembering her "movie" with as much detail as possible.

Connie's first attempt at this new type of lesson was a good one. Remember that just like her you are to choose a Focal Item, make a brief reconstruction of your picture from it, and then turn on the movie. Remember in as much detail as you can what happened and also what made the event arousing to you.

While engaging in your lessons this time, recollect your movie rather than give a physical description of the initial picture. Don't take too much time to mentally reconstruct your snapshot. However, keep in mind that it is important that you actually visualize your snapshot before you proceed with the lesson. It is critical that you have a precise starting point (and for now the *same* starting point) when beginning your recollection of the event. When you recall the event itself, remember not only the physical aspects of the event, but also in as much detail as possible what feelings and thoughts you had as it was happening. I want you to do the lesson a couple of times to familiarize yourself with how you can turn your snapshot into a movie.

After you become familiar with this procedure, pay special attention to what the "movie" actually looks like before getting involved in its emotional aspects. It is perfectly natural to have feelings creep in when you are thinking about your movie. In fact, that's great. That's exactly what I want you to experience when you think about your "movie." Often when this happens you'll find that your mind will be directed emotionally, and as a result many times you will not complete the entire "movie." Again, that's great. However, I want you initially to recollect the "movie" in strong detail and in its entirety. Therefore, as you carry this out the first time or two, concentrate on what the "movie" looks like and how it physically unfolds. Do each lesson with that in mind until you have a vivid recollection of the entire event. Spaces are provided for you to write down thoughts and additional physical details. Do two to four lessons within ten minutes during each of the morning, afternoon, and evening for a total of thirty minutes a day.

Initial Movie Recollection Form

Additional Details

Lesson 1

____

____

____

____

____

____

Lesson 2

____

____

____

____

____

____

Lesson 3

____

____

____

____

____

____

At times while you are doing your lessons you'll notice the emergence of thoughts and feelings that had long been forgotten. This is normal. Most people don't usually put themselves into the position to remember events in great detail. As time passes even exciting memories or feelings will fade and be forgotten either forever or until some stimulus triggers their recollection. It is important that you write down these forgotten thoughts and feelings to help you reinforce the memories and make them a more permanent part of your recollection.

To illustrate this method, let's return to our sample case study: While doing her lessons, Connie at times remembered certain thoughts and feelings that were not present when she initially recollected the event. During one lesson, she remembered that while she and her boyfriend were making love in the dirt and mud, she was imagining how people in primitive days probably did the same thing. Then she remembered mentally playing with the word *dirty*: "I thought about being 'dirty,' and I thought about being a nasty little girl for doing this. I didn't care, and the more I thought about being nasty the more I acted that way. From that thought, my mind abandoned everything except for the heavy lust and passion…my actions literally became wild, unquenchable."

Upon completing this particular lesson she returned to her form and condensed her thoughts and feelings into a few key words: "Dirty little girl," "hot, wild-acting…primitive sex!…abandoned behavior and mind."

During another lesson she remembered that at one point while they were making love her arms were outstretched in the mud. She remembered how the mud tickled the back of her arms when she slid them back and forth above her head. Within moments, reservations gave way to the "different, smooth" feel that cuddled her. After completing this lesson she returned to her form and noted: "Mud, arms and mud…slimy, smooth, and strange…but nice, too."

During her lessons Connie became aware of another feeling that was strong when the event occurred but that had faded over time and eventually had been overshadowed by the more prominent feelings of the event. This phenomenon happens to most people. Usually it is caused by a lack of effort invested in remembering the event. In this case, Connie remembered that as they were beginning to make love she heard a car door slam. The sound had come from the front of the house. As she heard it, her heart leaped, and she felt a warm flush come over her. Thinking that someone had probably stopped by to visit her, she became terrified:

> "What if whoever it was noticed the front door open and became suspicious when no one answered? What if we were too loud, and they came around to the garden? Maybe if we stayed still and didn't make any noise, whoever it was would go away and we wouldn't get caught! I have to admit that the fear of getting caught suddenly evaporated when my boyfriend whispered in my ear, 'You're the most beautiful thing I've ever seen…I love you!' After that, the whole world could have been watching or blown up as far as I was concerned and it wouldn't have mattered. That is how incredibly intense it was."

Upon completing her lesson, Connie returned to the form and compressed her thoughts into a few key words: "Feeling terrified and excited at the same time…weird!…fear of being caught…butterflies in my stomach…and those he put in my heart!"

You may have noticed that Connie's Focal Item allowed her to construct the initial scene and start her "movie" at nearly the beginning of her story, as she remembers it. Your recollection of a particular event is laid out in a fashion similar to that of the movies that you watch every day. A movie usually has a beginning, a middle, and an end and is played out in a sequence of individual scenes. So does your recollection of an event and indeed the event itself.

Connie went over her previous exercises, picking out a second Focal Item from the same scene in her "movie." When she visualized the scene this time, what stood out most in her mind was an image of herself from the back, as she was on her hands and knees. The Focal Item she visualized was the image of how she thought she looked to her boyfriend when he first came into the garden and saw her working there.

As you make the jump from one scene to another, a good way to think about it is to imagine that your movie is being played in a VCR. In this case, when you insert the videotape and press the "play" button, you start the movie in the middle of the story. It is an interesting scene, so you decide to watch it a while. After the interesting scene is over, you push "rewind" to restart the movie at the beginning.

Making this jump requires deliberately ending one thought, and then actively visualizing a second one. As you visualize the second thought, the initial mental image should be that of the Focal Item you had chosen earlier. Without your having previously selected a Focal Item, it is nearly impossible for you to control the direction and content of your thoughts.

We can see how Connie was able to manipulate her thoughts and to switch from one scene to another. When she finished her recollection of that particular scene, she put those immediate thoughts on hold. Then she quickly turned her attention to her second Focal Item. After visualizing it, she turned her movie back on:

> "I felt that the image I had about throwing my legs around him and holding him down on me were kind of like the end of the scene in Act II of my play. I thought this was a good place to stop thinking about what happened and switch to the beginning. So I started to visualize through my boyfriend's eyes how I looked on my knees, sitting up on my legs, the small outfit I had on, and my hair pulled back in a ponytail. The picture begins to move as I can see my image beginning to get larger, kind of like I was him walking closer to me, until my neck and my ear are the Focal Item. Then I can see his nose and mouth as he starts to kiss my neck and grab me from behind."

From there she continued with her recollection of the event.

Now that you understand the principle of this type of lesson, the schedule that you are to follow is similar to the one you used for the first series of lessons. But for this next series you will have a little more flexibility in the number of lessons you choose to do. However, a minimum number of lessons is required to achieve the desired results. Then, if you choose to increase your lesson time, all the better. You are to repeat each lesson set daily for four days. Upon completion, put your materials away for at least one day, two at most, before continuing.

For the first day, the lessons involve your recollection of the "movie" itself. You should make a special effort to limit your recollection to the physical description, leaving out any emotional component. Follow this approach to establish a good routine and an accurate and detailed remembrance of the event. As I have said, until you have become familiar with the story line and details of your movie, feeling any emotions while initially trying to remember the event might cause your mind to wander, hindering a clear and concise remembrance.

After you have completed the first day's lessons, carry out the remainder of the lessons in the normal fashion. This time include any feelings that you associate with your recollection. The rest of the lesson sets are to be done as stated earlier, that is, for three days, making a total of four days for this first lesson series.

- **When you have finished this series, take a break for one or two days before returning to it.**

Now let's proceed. As before, if the Focal Item that you used in the first series allowed you to start at the beginning of the story, your next Focal Item should be from the middle or end of the story. It is important to remember in selecting a new Focal Item that each subsequent selection should come from a different scene than the one before and that each scene chosen should represent a different moment within the story.

After you have chosen your new Focal Item, turn to the Final Movie Recollection Form that follows. It is also in the Workbook Section. In each form write down items or feelings that were forgotten or not included or new items that were remembered in your mental "movie." Do a minimum of three sets of lessons a day: one set during each of the morning, afternoon, and evening, devoting ten minutes to each lesson set. Do these lesson sets for three days. Upon completing them, again take a break, this time for only one day before proceeding with the next series.

After you have concluded the second series, begin a third and then a fourth. Just as before, follow the outline, structure, and schedule of the previous series.

SCHEDULE

First lesson series: Do a ten-minute lesson set, made up of two to four lessons, three times a day—morning, afternoon, and evening—for a total minimum of thirty minutes a day. Rest one day.

Second lesson series: Do a ten-minute lesson set, made up of two to four lessons, three times a day—morning, afternoon, and evening—for a total minimum of thirty minutes a day. Rest one day.

Third lesson series: Do a ten-minute lesson set, made up of two to four lessons, done three times a day—morning, afternoon, and evening—for a total minimum of thirty minutes a day. Rest one day.

Fourth lesson series: Do a ten-minute lesson set, made up of two to four lessons, done three times a day—morning, afternoon, and evening—for a total minimum of thirty minutes a day. Then stop.

Final Movie Recollection Form

Lesson 1 (Morning)

Items or feelings forgotten or not included during your movie recollection:

1.

2.

3.

New items or feelings remembered during your movie recollection:

1.

2.

3.

Lesson 2
Items or feelings forgotten or not included during your movie recollection:

1.

2.

3.

New items or feelings remembered during your movie recollection:

1.

2.

3.

Final Movie Recollection Form

Lesson 1 (Afternoon)

Items or feelings forgotten or not included during your movie recollection:

1.

2.

3.

New items or feelings remembered during your movie recollection:

1.

2.

3.

Lesson 2

Items or feelings forgotten or not included during your movie recollection:

1.

2.

3.

New items or feelings remembered during your movie recollection:

1.

2. ____

____

____

____

____

____

3. ____

____

____

____

____

____

Final Movie Recollection Form

Lesson 1 (Evening)

Items or feelings forgotten or not included during your movie recollection:

1. ____

____

____

____

____

____

2. ____

____

____

____

____

3.

New items or feelings remembered during your movie recollection:

1.

2.

3.

Lesson 2

Items or feelings forgotten or not included during your movie recollection:

1.

2.

3.

New items or feelings remembered during your movie recollection:

1.

2.

3.

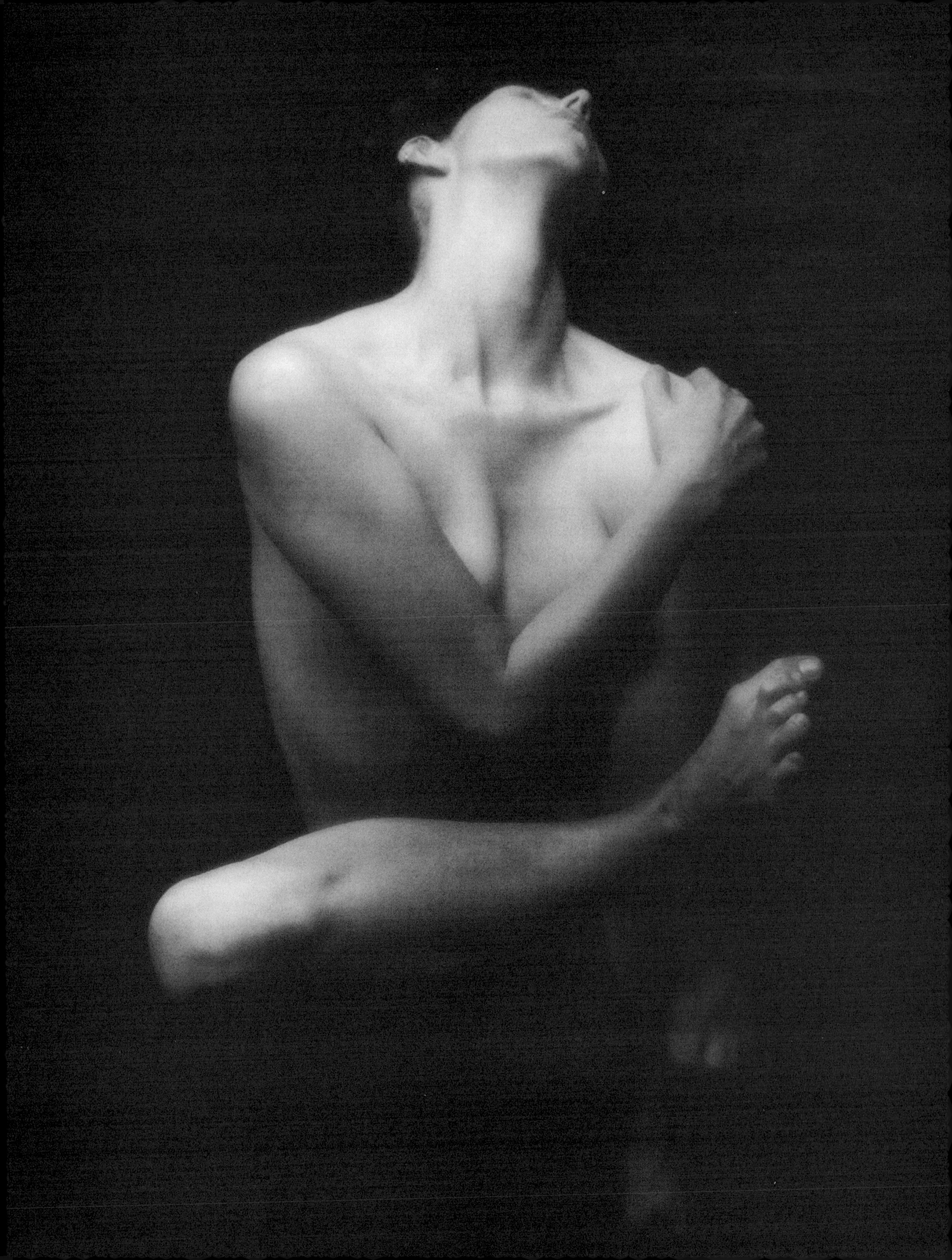

7

Chapter Seven

Flights of Fantasy

In searching for arousing material to use in your therapy, do not overlook the world of fantasy and your own fertile imagination, although for your first set of lessons I would prefer that you choose an event from real life. But if you are unable to recall anything arousing enough from your own past, you can use fantasies. They can be an excellent source.

In choosing a fantasy it is important that you choose your favorite—the one you find most arousing. Next, you will need to bring it into focus. Then you will need to give it a story line. And because by their nature most fantasies are incomplete, remembered ambiguously, or riddled with unrelated scenes, you may also need to give some thought to framing your fantasy with a beginning, a middle, and an end. Also, because a fantasy is usually visualized in a vague manner, you will need to clarify as many details as possible.

When someone visualizes a fantasy, even though she may be able to recall other parts of it, her initial recollection is of one or two main scenes. These main scenes usually represent the core of the fantasy.

Assuming that you now have a clear mental image of your fantasy, let's focus on your fantasy's story line. As I have mentioned, you need to turn your fantasy into a complete story. In doing so, you may need to expand on and embellish it, possibly creating new scenes to make it complete.

For example, if the main scene in your fantasy is that of you and Kevin Costner making love alongside a cabana on the beach, in completing the story you first need to ask yourself how the two of you got to that point—that is, how and where the two of you met and what happened that led to your making love on that particular beach. I know that right now you might be thinking: "Who cares how we got to that point?" But trust me, these details are important.

Then ask yourself questions such as who kissed whom first, how, and why. Who undressed whom, how, and why? Also, what was said between the two of you, if anything? Then, after you have developed, or recalled, the events leading to your principal scene, you need to give your story an ending. For example, when the two of you finished making love did you just lie there, did you talk, did you go for a swim, or get up, get dressed, and walk away?

After you have completed your story it is important that you write it down. I don't want you to turn your fantasy into a detailed novel, but rather into an outline of the order and direction that your story takes as you note things that stand out as you recall the story. Take some time now and fill out the following:

INITIAL FANTASY RECOLLECTION

Beginning

Middle

End

Let's examine the favorite fantasy of a woman named Francine. Hers involves herself, her husband, and another woman. Here is the initial description of her fantasy:

FRANCINE'S FANTASY

"My husband and I were out to dinner with a good friend, Roxanne, and after having too much to drink, we ended up at our house to continue our partying. After a few more drinks we decided to put on a fashion show with clothes that Roxanne had in her car (she was to model lingerie the next day). Well, things got a little crazy, and the three of us wound up making love in every way you could think of. For the rest of the weekend!"

As you probably can tell, this description is not ready to be used for her Solid Therapy lessons.

The next step is to give your fantasy a little more reality by fleshing it out, so to speak, with details. First, pick out one favorite scene. It's best that you choose the one that you find most arousing and that you think of most often when you recall your fantasy. Choose some Focal Items and list them in the blanks that follow. Turning your fantasy into a complete story is an important step in giving it the type of realism needed to get the most from it.

Take some time now and fill out the following.

SECOND FANTASY RECOLLECTION

____

____

Focal Items:

____

____

1. ______________________________________

____

____

____

____

____

2. ______________________________

____

____

____

3. ______________________________

____

____

____

____

After Francine revised her fantasy several times, here is the final version. The first part of her story is an actual occurrence, from which her fantasy springs:

"My husband and I had been out to dinner with a good friend of his, Roxanne, who had become a good friend of mine as well. We just finished a great meal and were polishing off our second bottle of wine when Roxanne said she had to leave, mumbling something about having to get up early the next day. After the customary hugs and pecks good-bye, we sat back down to enjoy an after-dinner drink, not that we needed one. He was telling me how sexy I looked and that he liked the way he could clearly see my nipples through my blouse, adding that he wasn't the only one who noticed my seeming arousal. I just kind of laughed, saying that I was glad at least somebody noticed. Then I said I was sure that he noticed Roxanne falling out of her blouse and that even I could see that she was obviously excited about something.

"'You really like her,' he said with a slight smugness. 'Of course,' I answered, 'she's really nice, we get along well, and I think she's fun to talk to.' 'No! That's not what I meant,' he interrupted. 'I mean, you really like her, don't you? I've seen the way you look at her.' I didn't think I felt those things about her…although at times I would feel a little twinge when we would touch or kiss hello or good-bye, but I never thought of it as being sexual…maybe it was! He went on, 'That's OK, I think it's cute you have a crush on her. I really wouldn't mind it that much if you did anything with her, just as long as you don't fall in love with her and leave me.'

"I knew he had to see how red my face had become, but that didn't slow him down at all. He kept commenting on how sexy I looked and went on and on about what Roxanne had worn and how sexy she looked. Finally I decided to jump in and agreed that she looked really hot! That seemed to shut him up for the moment. During the silence I saw him slowly lower his gaze to my chest. I knew he could see how hard my nipples had become with all the sexy talk. He looked up and smiled at me with a searching look in his eyes.

"Almost from the very start of our relationship, I knew that one of Michael's favorite fantasies was the possibility of bringing another person into our bed. It didn't take long for me to find the idea of another woman and myself kissing and touching as exciting as he probably did. But even in the heat of passion when the scary desire would surface in me, I was too embarrassed to bring it up. Michael has always been a considerate person, and when I never seemed to show an interest in doing something with another woman, he stopped bringing it up—much to my dismay.

"So it became one of those things that I purposely seldom thought about and definitely never verbalized. But now here I was talking to my husband about how sexy I thought another woman was, to his as well as my own disbelief. I kept commenting on her obvious attributes, and when I mentioned I thought it might be exciting to run my hands over her cute little butt, I could see him giving me another searching look. I was feeling no pain, and my diminishing inhibitions and building excitement only fueled my brazenness. So I decided to tell him when Roxanne and I hugged and kissed good-bye, I felt her hand touch the side of one of my breasts, and her tongue slipped between my lips and touched my teeth. This revelation seemed to bring a pensive look over his face…then, after a moment, 'So, what did you think of that?' he inquired, looking deeply into my eyes. 'I don't really know,' I responded. 'I kind of liked it, I guess.'

"He seemed to be even more quiet after my last comment; quiet, that is, until we got home. Once there, we had one of the wildest times I can remember. That night we felt freer and more uninhibited than ever. There was a lot more sexy talk, and we did a few things we never did before. After that night, I thought surely the subject would have come up, and I really wanted it to, but it didn't.

"But it's at the restaurant that my fantasy begins. Roxanne had just left, and we were sitting when suddenly I felt a pair of hands caress my shoulders. I turned my head quickly only to find myself staring into Roxanne's beautiful blue eyes. She informed us that as she started to drive off, she received a call on her car phone telling her that her morning appointment had been canceled, so she thought she would come back to celebrate!

"Roxanne is a model, and she told us that she was scheduled to do a layout for a lingerie company, and she had a suitcase full of things that she was to wear for the next morning's shoot. During our conversation, she would take every opportunity to touch me and tell me how beautiful I was. It seemed innocent enough at first; however, at one point she rested her hand on my thigh and said while looking into my eyes that I was unbelievably sexy and had a much better body than she did. This reaction caused by 'another woman' made me both excited and embarrassed. I was hoping Michael didn't notice how flushed I'd become, but when I glanced over at him, his smile said everything. She insisted that I should be the one to model the lingerie, and to prove her point she suggested that we go back to our house and try some of the clothes on. She told us that Michael should take a few Polaroids of her and me wearing different outfits, and that we should let Michael be the judge as to who looked best. Hearing this suggestion, my husband had us both in the car and home before you could translate *ménage à trois.*

"Once home, Michael took our drink orders, and Roxanne and I dragged the suitcase upstairs to get ready for our show. There were all kinds of things, from conservative to ultra-sexy. I chose a midthigh, white silky robe, and she selected a pair of blue paisley Bermuda-style silk shorts with matching camisole. I was a little nervous as we hurried down to the den to show Michael what we put on. I had worn sexy lingerie before, but not in a situation like this, so I was a little worried he would think I looked out of character. Silly thought! His low moan of appreciation was all I needed to know how he felt.

"I decided to go first and moved to the center of the room while Michael went to get the Polaroid and our camcorder, saying that he wanted to record this for posterity. Roxanne began to direct me into different provocative poses. I let the thin robe fall open every chance I got, making sure they could see I had nothing on underneath. It felt great but also scary to be showing off my body to someone else other than my husband.

"After several shots it was Roxanne's turn. I took over the camcorder. As Roxanne began to pose I realized I was disappointed with her selection. Although she looked great (she always does), deep down inside I was hoping I would get to see more of her lovely body than her outfit allowed. However, her posing was unbelievable. She really knew what to do with her body, and even though you couldn't actually see anything through the material, she gave the impression she had nothing on!

"When she finished she grabbed my hand, and we ran up the stairs giggling, like little kids playing dress-up in their mother's clothes. A feeling began to wash over me that I couldn't recognize. It was, however, one I had felt many times before when I was with Roxanne. When we reached the bedroom Roxanne turned to me and said, 'This is so much fun getting dressed up for you. It's like I'm getting ready for a date!' That was it!...What I had been feeling all those times, just like now, was like I was on a date...a date with a woman!

"Before I could sort out everything going on in my mind I heard Roxanne say, 'This time I think we should pick out each other's outfit.' Right away I thought, 'Great! Now I'll get my chance to select something that will let me see as much of her beautiful body as I want.' But it didn't hit me until I saw what she was handing me that perhaps this was exactly what she had in mind for me. She picked out the very outfit I was going to choose for her. A short, white minipush-up, half-cupped bustier with matching garter and stockings, and the panties were see-through lace that rose high on the hips. I'm sure she could see the stunned look on my face as I deftly accepted her 'offering.' 'OK, where's mine?' she asked, breaking my trance.

"I turned quickly to look over the selections. I was determined to choose one that was even more revealing than the one she picked out for me. I zeroed in on the perfect thing. It screamed sex! There was a five- or six-inch-wide, plain, soft, black cotton garter belt, with wide straps hanging from it, which attached to opaque black thigh-high stockings. And the black cotton G-string was so small it didn't seem to be made for an adult. The bra was strapless and made of the same plain, wide, black cotton, narrowing only under each breast, exposing nearly everything. Snatching it up, I turned to see Roxanne grinning at my selection.

"I was waiting for her to go into the dressing room to change, like she did before. But it became quite obvious that she had no intention of doing so. Still too shy to blatantly strip in front of her, even though I wished I had the nerve, I turned slightly around and sheepishly began to change, pretending she wasn't there. Could I really let her see me like this, knowing I was dressed like this for her? I knew as I slipped into my shoes that the time had come; I had to gather up enough courage to turn and face her. So with all the determination I could muster, I did. But the moment I looked into her beautiful blue eyes, any unexpected courage I may have discovered just jumped right out the window! I thought to myself, I can't believe it—here I was virtually naked in front of Roxanne, and by the look on her face that's exactly how she wanted me to be. I was too scared to make the first move, but I was hoping for something to happen, yet at the same time trying to think of how I could get Michael up here. As often as I had thought about this, I realized a good part of my excitement would come from having my husband actually watching me touch, kiss, and make love with another woman.

"But suddenly, without a word, she just turned and went into the bathroom to change, leaving me there charged with frustration. I couldn't understand why she went into the other room until the door swung open, and there stood the most beautiful creature I had ever seen in my life. The black stockings and wide garter with its wide straps framed her beautiful hips, drawing my eyes to her exposed flesh. The black pumps made her legs look even longer, if that were possible. And the tiny G-string hid literally nothing…it took my breath away. But it was the sight of her exposed breasts that made my heart actually ache! Just the thought that I might have a chance to actually touch them and maybe get to feel them with my lips almost made me cry from wanting them so badly. She walked toward me as if it were a dream. Reaching out her hand, she let it stop softly on my cheek. 'Let's go downstairs, before I change my mind and keep you all to myself,' I heard her say, breaking the spell once more.

"I felt her hand touch the small of my back and slide to my waist as she walked around me, giving me a chance, for the first time, to see her beautiful butt. I knew I was supposed to follow her, but my legs were literally too weak to move. I didn't know what to do about it, but I didn't have to worry for long. Because as she passed the bed Roxanne hopped up on it to adjust her stockings. Patting the space next to her, she asked if I could give her a hand. So I sat next to her to help her out. I could feel her move her thigh against mine as I leaned over her to help adjust the garter's snap. And as if in a tunnel I heard someone say, 'You're so beautiful…I'm scared…but I'm even more excited,' she breathed. As I straightened up, my face came to rest only inches from hers. Then I heard myself softly say, 'Roxanne, my heart is pounding in my throat.' As if looking straight down into my soul she responded, 'I don't want you to do anything you don't want to.' I was going to tell her the same thing, but before I could her mouth was on mine! The heat rising in my body was incredible as I felt her bare arms encircle my body…"

Francine's story is well organized and very detailed. Hers would be the ideal. However, you do not have to be as descriptive as she was to benefit from your fantasy. The techniques that you have learned in the previous chapters will help to make your fantasy workable.

If you are not as able as Francine to visualize your story clearly, do not hesitate to use a Visual Subsidy, as described in Chapter Eight. If you decide to use a Visual Subsidy, my advice is to choose a photograph or picture that closely resembles the mental image you have of your fantasy. But it does not have to be an identical representation of your mental image. Details can vary; for example, your Visual Subsidy might depict a daytime scene, whereas your fantasy might take place at night. The presence of people in your Visual Subsidy is irrelevant as well; some people find them distracting, whereas others say they help in embellishing their fantasy. What is important is that you have a feeling of connection between your Visual Subsidy and your fantasy.

After you have selected a Visual Subsidy, review Chapter Eight for instructions on how to turn your subsidy into a usable format.

Fantasies are great! Do not be afraid to use your wonderful mind and have a great time! Fill in the following as outlined in Chapters Four and Six.

FINAL FANTASY SNAPSHOT RECOLLECTION FORM

Lesson 1

Items forgotten or not included during your recollection:

1. ______________________________

____

____

____

____

____

2. ______________________________

____

____

____

____

____

____

3.

New items remembered during your recollection:

1.

2.

3.

Lesson 2
Items forgotten or not included during your recollection:

1.

2.

3.

New items remembered during your recollection:

1.

2.

3.

Lesson 3
Items forgotten or not included during your recollection:

1.

2.

3.

New items remembered during your recollection:

1.

2.

3.

Lesson 4
Items forgotten or not included during your recollection:

1.

2.

3.

New items remembered during your recollection:

1.

2.

3.

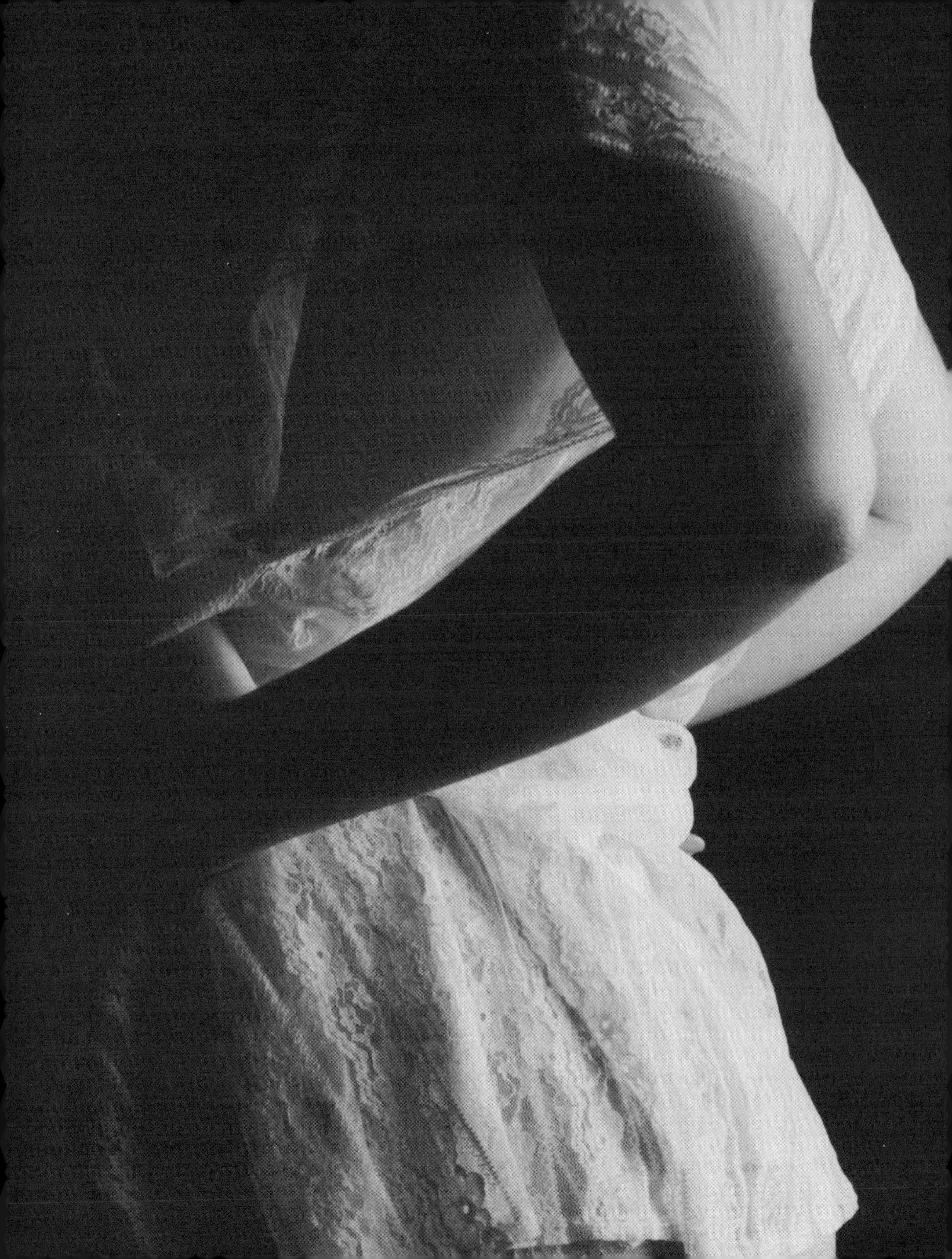

8

Chapter Eight

Seeing Is Believing

Sight is the sense from which people most commonly receive arousing stimuli. In this chapter we will demonstrate how you can use sight to improve your imperfect recollection of arousing events. How? Through the use of a Visual Subsidy. A Visual Subsidy is a picture or photograph that helps you to recall, reconstruct, and even embellish an event.

Often when you are participating in an event, you do not notice the surrounding details or do not want to take time to notice them. And we are all aware of what time later can do to our recollection of that event: Either we forget the event altogether, or at the very least we forget numerous details of it. Thus, even though we may retain strong feelings about the event, our memory may be narrowed to just its basics—the bare bones. I have found that although this type of narrowed memory has great potential for arousing us, often we can't use it quickly and easily.

But a Visual Subsidy can help us to put some flesh on those bare bones. To clarify, I will highlight another case study.

CASE STUDY OF LORI

Lori, thirty-three, had always remembered a particular event from her final year of college. The event was one of the most exciting of her life. However, the intervening years had taken their toll, dulling the sharp edges of her recollection. What she remembered of the event she still found very exciting even after all those years, but her memory had been narrowed to just the basics. At our first interview, Lori stated that she seldom thought of the event spontaneously. In fact, she often had to made a conscious effort to remember it, even though she still found it exciting. Lori also said that nothing she would subconsciously recognize would elicit her recollection of the event. Here is Lori's recollection:

> "It was in the summer of my last year at interior design school, and at the time I was dating this really handsome guy. His parents were really nice, very well educated, and had a lot of money. About midsummer I planned a trip to visit him at their home, which was huge and really beautiful. Well, very late one afternoon after we had played tennis, I was up in this gorgeous bathroom getting ready to take a shower when my boyfriend came in. I told him he should get out of there because we might get caught. He said that he'd been going crazy all summer and couldn't wait any longer and wanted to do something right there. I told him that he would just have to go back to playing with himself because I wasn't going to do anything there. He didn't give up, and we kept talking until things got a little different. Anyway, I wound up doing something in the tub, while telling him that he could only watch. That's when things got really sexy."

Even when pressed, Lori was unable to elaborate much more. Because this event still held intense feelings for her, we decided that she should use a Visual Subsidy. After searching through various materials, she found a photograph in a magazine devoted to bedroom and bathroom remodeling. The bathroom in the photograph was very similar to the actual bathroom where her event took place.

Your first goal for this chapter is to choose your own Visual Subsidy by finding a picture that relates to a particular event that you find sensual or erotic. That picture, as your Visual Subsidy, will be used as your snapshot in forthcoming lessons. Therefore, your picture should have some relationship to, and remind you of, that particular event.

Visual Subsidies can include photographs and pictures in books, magazines, and paintings and images from movies and TV, but photographs and pictures seem to work best. I have found that women get better results with fashion and travel magazines. This may be because these magazines are aimed at women and their particular needs and desires. The advertisements seem to be even more enticing than their editorial layouts.

Your selection does not have to be erotic or sexual in itself. On the contrary, it can be very subtle. Often people can recall and embellish an arousing event from the most innocent Visual Subsidy, such as everyday magazine advertisements and TV commercials. In selecting your picture, keep in mind one of two criteria. Select a picture that represents an experience that has actually occurred to you. This picture will help you re-create that particular experience. Or choose a picture that has little or no relationship to your experience but that you find particularly arousing. This photograph will expand your creative thoughts by making use of your imagination and fantasies.

For now, we will use a picture that represents an experience that has actually occurred to you. It does not have to be a perfect match, but it should be similar enough to remind you of that experience.

The next step is to re-create the scene where the actual experience took place in as much detail as possible.

Take some time now and fill out the following. Additional Visual Subsidy Snapshot Recollection Forms are in the Workbook Section that begins on page 159.

VISUAL SUBSIDY SNAPSHOT RECOLLECTION PART 1
Briefly describe your chosen event:

____

____

____

____

____

____

____

____

____

____

Just as before, you will re-create a snapshot or initial scene, from which you will begin your lessons. Only this time, you will use the Visual Subsidy instead of relying solely on your memory.

After you have chosen your Visual Subsidy, examine it closely. In the Workbook Section and in the spaces that follow here are three columns. The first column is to list the things about your Visual Subsidy that are similar to or identical to your recollection of the actual event. The second column is to list things that are in your Visual Subsidy but that are not in your recollection of the event. And the third column is to list things that are in your recollection of the event but that are not in your Visual Subsidy. I am sure that from the outset you will be aware of many similarities and differences between your Visual Subsidy and your recollection. Therefore, first write down the differences. As you begin, you will recall more details than you would have if you had attempted to recall them only mentally. The more details of the event that you are able to remember and write down, the more the Visual Subsidy will reinforce your memory of the event and increase your connections to it.

Take as much time as you need. And taking a breather to clear your mind may enhance your recollection.

VISUAL SUBSIDY SNAPSHOT RECOLLECTION PART 2

Like Items	Unlike Items	Missing Items

After you have completed this form, set aside your Visual Subsidy for a while, then return to it and review your material, making any last-minute additions. After you feel that your recollection and form are complete, we are ready to continue.

Returning to our case study, we find that after Lori completed the preceding process she was able to make these recollections:

> "It was the most marvelous bathroom; two of the walls and almost all of the woodwork was done up in various shades of grayish greens. One wall, which had a quaint window in the middle of it, was covered with a green and white English floral print. A section of another wall, by one of the doorways (there were two), was plastered differently and was painted with a faded fresco, a watercolor vine scene. There was a lightly stained oak floor in the room partially covered with an antique-looking floral-illustrated Kurdistan-type carpet, done in faded burgundies, mauves, beiges, pinks, and greens. There was a large closed-in tub with recessed lighting. The walls around the tub were made of three large forest green panels against wide lighter green framework. On one corner of the tub there was a large white seashell containing several natural sponges. The room was very large, and the broad mirrors around the tub made it look even larger, but yet it had a very safe and comfortable, cozy feeling.
>
> "The room had many pictures, arranged in twos and threes, both in columns and singularly. I remember one that appeared old and was of two kids washing themselves

in a small creek. Most of the pictures had a bathroom motif. There were also a couple depicting what I believe were old European cities, and my favorite was a framed tapestry, slightly faded, portraying an old English bathroom. Against one wall there was a large floor-to-ceiling vanity, done in the same shades of greens and white. There was a white marble counter and white porcelain sink with matching fixtures. Above the sink was a recessed beveled mirror, neighbored on either side by ceiling-high open shelves displaying decorative objects: beautiful glass canisters of different sizes, labeled with black and gold-leaf lettering and designs, containing different bath powders and soaps. A crystal and brass clock, a Roman bust, a baby panda, and a penguin figure. A handful of different colored seashells, four or five antique silver picture frames with old photographs of people, several bottles made of crystal, glass, silver, et cetera, containing perfumes and oils, and a few antique books. On the counter was a small crystal vase filled with large pink and red roses, fully open. Next to the vanity was an Adam gilt wood open armchair with an antique, faded, dark green, fringed floral-printed cushion. In one corner there was a large plaster floor vase filled with vibrant pink and white hydrangeas.

"The other side of the room was a little sitting area, complete with a makeup table arranged in front of a large window, decorated with a dark green and mauve printed valance, slightly pinched and with lively green, white, and rose floral-printed drapes, pulled back with a green tie. Underneath the drapes I remembered noticing Scottish lace sheers, with Scalamandre glass-beaded trim. There was also an off-white, channel-back chair and ottoman. The chair had rolled arms with fan pleats and a high kick-pleat flounce. Around the table and chair were three small needlework pillows..."

Do you notice the dramatic contrast between Lori's first description and one she made with the aid of a Visual Subsidy? This is not the exception. In fact, you will find that when using a Visual Subsidy, once-forgotten details are defined with new clarity. Whether the details in Lori's new description were accurate doesn't matter because the scene that Lori then described, with all its details, had been incorporated into her memory of the event, making her memory, in effect, fact. Continuing with Lori's recollection:

"I was visiting at his parents' house for a few days. It was a Friday, and I remember it being very cloudy and threatening to storm all afternoon, and we had just finished playing tennis with some of his friends at the country club. We had plans to go out to dinner with his parents and a couple of their friends that evening. When we got back to his house I had just enough time to take a quick nap and get ready. I told my boyfriend what I was going to do, and he suggested that he 'take a little nap with me.' We hadn't seen much of each other that summer, except in the beginning of it for one weekend before he started his summer job. And by this time I think it would have been a toss-up as to who was more horny. But even though I missed him a lot, I couldn't overcome the uneasiness I had about doing something in his parents' house, especially since most of his family were home by that time. I told him that I felt too uncomfortable to do anything there. But he kept pushing it. He would grab me and tell me things he wanted to do to me. He told me that he had been going crazy all summer without 'me and my hot little body.' But in spite of my really wanting to, I couldn't get the fear or uncomfortable feelings out of my mind.

"Finally I had to get firm with him and told him to 'chill out!' And if he was that horny he should just take care of it himself. I didn't mean to be so cruel, but I just couldn't do anything there. I left him sulking in the living room and went upstairs to crash out. I woke up about an hour later and went into the bathroom to take a shower and get ready. I was still a little groggy as I was undressing. As my mind began to clear, I started to remember parts of a dream I had while I was napping. I guess finally getting to see my boyfriend after such a long time, and all that touching and dirty talk, must have gotten to me more than I thought. I don't remember exactly what the dream was now, but I do remember that the more I thought about it, the more I was getting excited. I had taken off all my clothes except for my tennis skirt and was about to unzip that, too, when I couldn't stand it any longer, so I slipped one hand down inside my skirt instead of unzipping it and at the same time brought the other one up to my bare chest and began to touch myself. I could see myself in the mirror. Between my reflection and what was going through my mind, I was distracted, to say the least.

"As my mind continued to wander I gradually began to sense the presence of someone else in the room. Still looking in the mirror, my eyes suddenly focused on the figure of someone sitting on the edge of the bathtub. It was my boyfriend! Startled, I spun around and quickly pulled my other hand up to my chest, trying to cover myself up the best I could. I started to yell at him for frightening me and for being there. My scream and sudden move scared him, too, because he jumped up quickly and started to stammer incoherently. I was really mad and asked him what the hell he thought he was doing sneaking up and spying on me like that. He was frantically trying to calm me down, telling me he was sorry but it wasn't his fault. He said that the one door was open, and he just walked in not knowing I was up yet, let alone in the bathroom.

"The bathroom did have the two doors, and I realized he was telling the truth—I didn't lock the one he came in through. I started to calm down, but the more I did, the more embarrassed I became, thinking he was actually watching me do something so private like that. I could see he noticed my embarrassment, as a grin came over his face. Then he said, 'I see I'm not the only one who has those kinds of problems.' With that I started to get even more embarrassed. He kept it up, asking me all kinds of things like, he didn't know I did anything like that, and did I do it a lot, and did I do it different ways, and what I liked the best, et cetera. I was so embarrassed by then I really don't remember exactly what he was saying. He seemed to be taking pleasure in my predicament and began teasing me mercilessly. There was no way to get out of this gracefully, so I decided to do what I knew would work best—fight back!

"I asked him what his problem was...did he feel threatened knowing that he could be replaced so easily? Well, that shut him up in a hurry. Now, I had him on the ropes, and I wasn't going to let him go so easily. Then I asked him in a snotty tone, 'What's the matter, didn't you like what you saw?' In a now-timid manner he hesitated for a moment, then said softly, 'I've never seen you look so beautiful.' Some very quiet moments passed before I heard myself saying, 'Would you like to see what I really like to do?' He looked dazed but managed to daftly shake his head yes. I couldn't believe it was me talking. I don't know what got into me; all I did know...I was excited as hell!

"I told him to pull up one of the chairs and watch! As he did, I moved over to the tub and turned the water on. I glanced over my shoulder to see the look on his face as I slipped my skirt down around my ankles, then stepped into the tub. I lay down and put my feet up against the wall, placing one foot on either side of the faucet. Then I slid my bottom forward until what I wanted was directly under the running water, and..."

Again, this passage shows you the enormous contrast between Lori's first recollection and what she was able to recall after using a Visual Subsidy. Although Lori may have been more adept at expressing herself than most people are, that isn't what is important. What is important is the results that people get from a Visual Subsidy.

After you have completed the preceding exercise, reviewing your Visual Subsidy and filling in your form, you have essentially created—or, more precisely, *re-created*—a snapshot. This snapshot is very much like the ones that you have created previously, with the obvious exception that this one is partly a visual snapshot and partly a mental snapshot instead of solely a mental one.

The next step is for you to transfer the visual snapshot to a mental one. You need to do this because in everyday life you will not always be able to grab your Visual Subsidy every time you want to become aroused.

The lessons for this next section are similar to the others. They are divided into three hours: one in the morning, one it the afternoon, and one in the evening. Each hour is divided into four parts, and each part represents one lesson. However, you will notice that there is much more space available for writing.

This is how each lesson should be attempted: First, examine your Visual Subsidy and your list of additional details. When finished, put the material aside, and wait for ten to fifteen minutes before returning to the lesson. When you return, in the space provided, jot down—from memory—a few of the major details of your photograph. Do not copy them directly from the Visual Subsidy or from the list, but rather get them from the mental picture that you have re-created. When you have finished, compare your photograph and your mental picture, making sure that you are aware of the things you might have left out. You may have noticed that your recollection of the Visual Subsidy is a little disorganized. This is normal.

- **Now take your time and fill out the following, giving a more detailed description of your chosen event:**

VISUAL SUBSIDY SNAPSHOT RECOLLECTION PART 3
Recollection:

Like Items	Unlike Items	Missing Items

Now that you know the basics, select one detail from the Visual Subsidy scene, which you will use as your Focal Item in reconstructing your mental picture. After you have chosen your Focal Item, while looking at your Visual Subsidy and list, begin your second lesson by focusing on that item. From there, widen your view of the photograph by adding more of the details from both your Visual Subsidy and list until you have completely constructed your picture. When you have completed that, again set the material aside for ten to fifteen minutes before returning to it. Then, using the spaces provided, begin to reconstruct your mental snapshot from memory. This time begin by creating in your mind an image of your Focal Item. Then from that point, mentally reconstruct your mental snapshot. For these first few lessons, it is vital that you not only devote enough time to make yourself familiar with your Visual Subsidy in general, but also that you become familiar with and include as many details as possible. This seeming preoccupation with details is essential. It will drastically widen your ability not only to associate items with your principal memory, but also to discover and use their often compelling nature. These details will be able to evoke a sensual response in connection with your memory of an event, and eventually many of them will be able to evoke the desired response on their own.

After you have completed your mental reconstruction, review your Visual Subsidy and list. Make a note of what you forgot to include in your mental recollection of the Visual Subsidy scene. Each time you encounter a detail that was not included in your memory, write it down. Also, if while recalling your snapshot you remember any new details that were not previously contained in your picture, write them down. Now fill out the following:

COMPLETE VISUAL SUBSIDY SNAPSHOT RECOLLECTION FORM
Lesson 1
Focal Items:

____

____

Recollection:

____

____

____

____

____

____

____

____

____

____

____

____

Complete your next lesson in the same manner as the first lesson: by first looking over your Visual Subsidy and list, using your Focal Item as a starting point and impressing on your mind the entire scene. Set aside the material for the same amount of time, then return and begin with a mental starting point. After you have completed it, review your Visual Subsidy and list, make a comparison, and write in the spaces that follow the details that you had forgotten to include. Complete the lessons in this manner for the next two days.

Like Items	**Unlike Items**	**Missing Items**

The remainder of the lessons in this series are to be completed in the following manner:

Instead of beginning with an examination of your Visual Subsidy and list, begin by making a mental image of your Focal Item. Then reconstruct your mental snapshot. After completing the reconstruction, take out your Visual Subsidy and list and review them, noting the things that were not included in your recollection. Also, be aware of any new material that comes to mind.

Continue your lessons in this manner for the next five days, carrying out a minimum of two to four lessons of fifteen minutes each (one lesson set). Complete at least one lesson set during each of the morning, afternoon, and evening.

When these five days of lessons have been concluded, rest for one or two days. Then do a new series of lessons. These lessons will be carried out in the same manner except that for each day's lessons you are to select a new Focal Item from which to begin. Do these lessons for five days. After you have completed this series, you should have used at least eight Focal Items. If you wish to continue with this lesson, please do. The more you do, the more you will benefit. Also, at this time you may want to start this lesson series anew, using a new event and Visual Subsidy.

Following is an outline that reviews this lesson series. For each day of lessons, follow the lesson plan labeled "Visual Subsidy Forms" in the Workbook Section. Each day's lesson is divided into three parts—morning, afternoon, and evening—and each time period is from fifteen minutes to one hour long.

SCHEDULE

Day one, first lesson series, first lesson: In the forms that follow, do the lessons as laid out—one lesson during each of the morning, afternoon, and evening. If you can do more than one lesson in the morning, great. And four would be ideal.

Examine your Visual Subsidy and list.

Choose a Focal Item.

Make a mental recollection and from memory write down on the proper form the major details.

Compare mental recollection with Visual Subsidy and list.

Note the differences on the form.

Days two through five, first lesson series: In the forms that follow, do as before but add at least one or two lessons during each of the morning, afternoon, and evening.

Examine your Visual Subsidy and list.

Make a mental recollection and from memory write down on the proper form the major details.

Compare mental recollection with Visual Subsidy and list.

Note the differences on the form.

Days six through twelve, second lesson series: In the forms that follow, do as for days one through five, but use a new Focal Item for each day's lessons.

When this has been completed, return to Chapter Four and continue with the remainder of your therapy, using this material for your lessons.

FINAL VISUAL SUBSIDY RECOLLECTION FORM

Lesson 1

Focal Item:

Recollection:

Like Items	Unlike Items	Missing Items

Lesson 2
Focal Item:

Recollection:

Like Items	Unlike Items	Missing Items

Lesson 3
Focal Item:

Recollection:

Like Items	Unlike Items	Missing Items

Lesson 4
Focal Item:

Recollection:

Like Items	Unlike Items	Missing Items

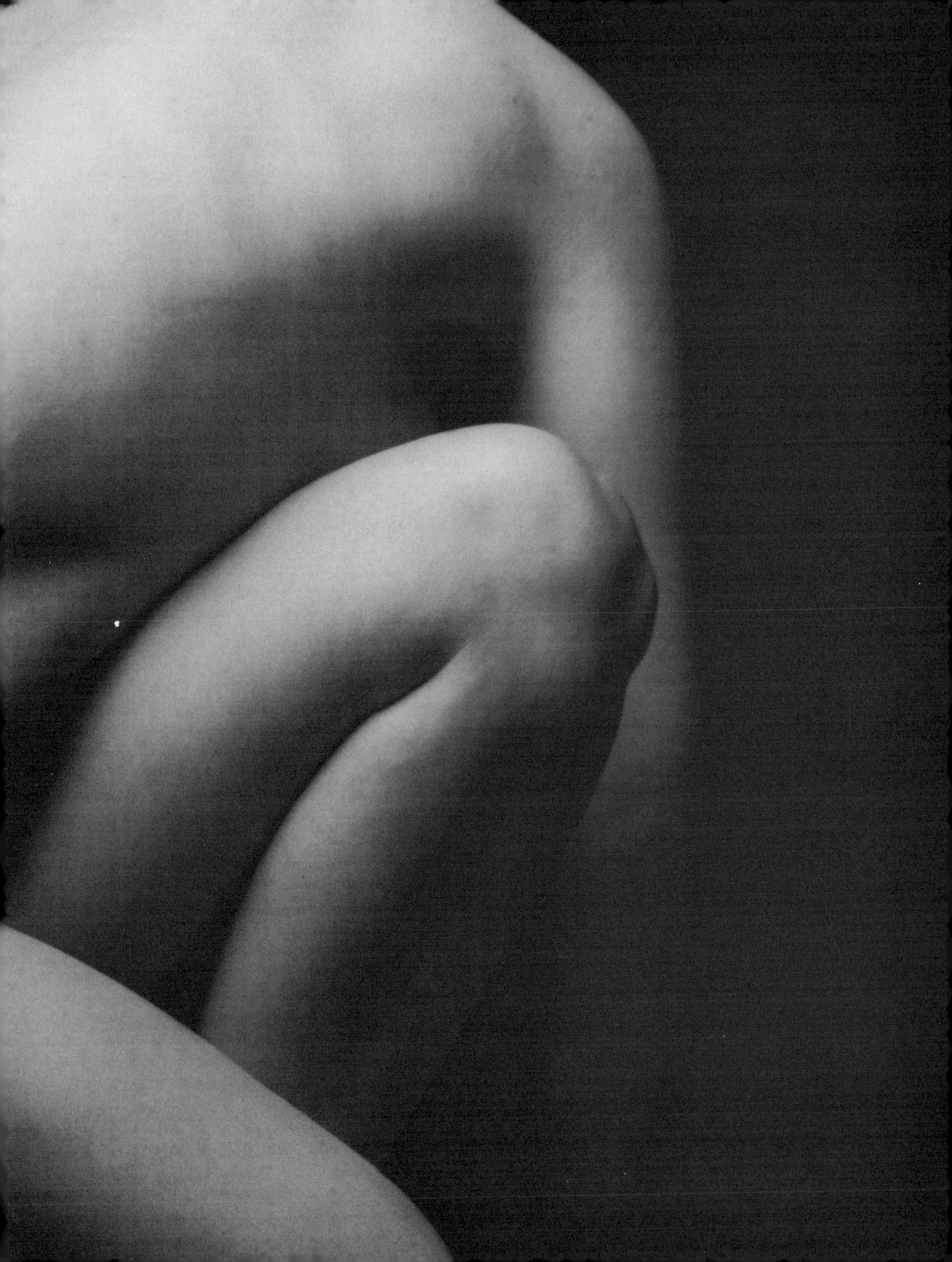

9

Chapter Nine

The Ears Have It

Sound is one of our strongest and most sensitive connections to the past. It can even rapidly alter a person's emotions without her being aware of it. Sound also has the power to elicit erotic feelings. And that's what we are most interested in. To channel that power for our lessons, you will need a tape player or CD player, earphones for privacy, and recordings of the songs or sounds that you have strong connections with.

This type of therapy is very beneficial, but it can also be cumbersome and inconvenient. It is important that you do not attempt this part of your therapy until you have a good working knowledge of Solid Therapy.

After you have gathered the sound equipment, let's begin. First, review the memories of events—not just arousing events—in your life that you associate with a particular song or sound. I am sure that you will become aware of many songs and sounds that remind you of experiences and that evoke a variety of emotions: happiness, sadness, nostalgia, excitement, and so forth. Then, as you recollect, pick out the songs and sounds that you associate with sensual events or feelings. You may be surprised, as most people are, to discover that you can associate quite a few songs and sounds with sensual situations. For now, I want you to write down, in the form labeled "Sound (Song) List," all the songs and sounds that remind you of something sensual. Next to each song and sound, write what it reminds you of. As an example, here's how a patient named Maddy responded:

MADDY'S LIST

Sound (Song) List

"Doing the Butt" (song)—Dance club, blasted, wild time, Bobby's place.

"Never Live Without You" (song)—Denver, mountains, freedom.

Tears for Fears (singing group)—California, nighttime, Highway 10, Denny's restaurant.
"Hotel California" (song)—San Diego, Hotel Coronado, dinner.
"Thunder and lightning"—Michael's place, bedroom balcony door open, up until 5 A.M.!
"Blowing winds"—Phoenix, Arizona, hot tub, nighttime.
Phil Collins, *Genesis* (singer, rock group)—Our house, den, surprise striptease.
Jet engines—Trip to California, hot day, pool, jets going over, champagne.
Michael Franks (songwriter)—Us lying in bed in my apartment on a cold December morning having toast and tea, Sunday paper, me with a small, white, lace and cotton teddy.
"I Feel the Earth Move" (song)—Palm Springs, earthquake while in bed, Riviera Hotel, and so forth.

• **Now it's your turn:**

Sound (Song) List

1. ______________________________

____

____

____

____

2. ______________________________

____

____

____

3. ______________________________

____

____

____

After Maddy completed her list, she was asked to go over it and pick a song or sound that she wanted to begin her first lesson with. Then, on the form labeled "Sound Snapshot Form 1" she wrote her selection—the Phil Collins song—in the space marked "Sound Focus." Then she was asked to write a short synopsis of the event in her memory and how the sound or song was connected to it.

MADDY'S SOUND FOCUS

SOUND SNAPSHOT FORM 1

Sound Focus: Phil Collins

Short Synopsis: "My boyfriend and I have had a very good sex life, or at least I think so. We used to talk about many things pertaining to sex and were pretty open about what we liked and some of our fantasies. Once when we were watching a movie on cable, he happened to make a comment about a girl that was doing a striptease during a bar scene. He said something like, 'Boy, you never do anything like that for me.' And I said, 'I never thought you liked that.' He responded by saying that he usually didn't, but the thought of me doing it was exciting to him. Getting a little interested, I asked him what he found exciting about it. He started by telling me what he didn't find exciting, like her movements were too jerky and the music was too fast.

"He then added that he didn't find the idea of a stranger taking off her clothes for people she didn't know especially exciting. I asked him teasingly, since he was such an 'expert,' how he thought it should be done. He looked at me and smiled. First of all, he said, it has to be done by someone that you really like. Just the thought of somebody you love standing in front of you, ready to take off their clothes for you, and knowing what it will probably lead to, is too much for me not to appreciate. He went on and added that the girl shouldn't dress up in something stupid like a cowboy costume, but rather she should have on something nice. I asked what he meant by 'nice,' and he said, 'nothing flashy, a nice blazer with a skirt or pants, or a nice evening gown. Something normal with unbelievably sexy lingerie on underneath.' Then he said something that really got my attention. He told me what he thought would be really exciting is if I stripped to the Phil Collins song *In the Air Tonight*. Obviously he had given this more thought than he was letting on.

"We let the subject drop, and neither of us brought it up again. Ever since then, whenever I heard a Phil Collins song or a Genesis record played on the radio, my mind would wander off and begin thinking about the conversation we had earlier. It didn't have to be the exact song; any one of their songs would prompt me to start getting more excited about actually doing a striptease.

"Finally, one day I decided that I really wanted to do it. The idea of exciting him was great, but I think I was more excited by the thought of actually doing it. When I was alone, I would flip through cable looking for programs that had strippers in them, then watch. I didn't like most of them, but there were a few things in their routines I thought were erotic, and those I would make mental notes of. I was a big fan of Phil Collins and already had a copy of that particular song. A couple of times I would put it on and watch myself in front of a mirror mimicking some of the movements, as well as making up some of my own I thought were sexy. I felt a little awkward at first, but that didn't last too long. It really got me excited! I was planning every detail so everything was perfect. Finally I was ready.

"It was a Friday. All day long my mind was like a bowl of guacamole. I had to work that day, but all I could think of was what I had planned for that evening. I could not believe I would soon be dancing in plain view, on display, doing a striptease. I had already set up the tape player in the den and had put on the long version of the song in order to give me all the time I wanted. We had made reservations at an upscale restaurant, so he arrived wearing a fabulous double-breasted suit. It was about eight o'clock, and I asked him to make a couple of drinks while I finished dressing. Meanwhile, I was putting on the finishing touches.

"My outfit consisted of a structured black and white small vine-printed evening jacket (which looked almost gray), a white silk soft-collared blouse, a low-cut, white cotton bodysuit (slightly transparent), a thin, delicate, lace bustier, and white, almost opaque arm gloves that started at my wrists and stopped at my elbows. You couldn't see the gloves under the jacket and blouse. The skirt was around midthigh and was of the opposite matching print of the jacket. Under that, I had on white stretch pants and white stockings that had an 'S' pattern down the back of my leg, 'S' for *slut*! The stockings were attached to a matching lace garter belt and a pair of beautiful light floral lace panties. I wore a pair of conservative gray heels and accessorized with multiple strands of long pearls, bracelets, earrings, et cetera. I wanted to have plenty to take off. That is where my idea to wear more than one outfit started. If anything, it was different. I wanted this to be better than any fantasy and to definitely be a performance to remember.

"From the first glance you couldn't tell what I had planned. When I got to the den he was sitting on the couch watching television. I walked in and shut off the TV without saying a word. He started to say something, but I cut him off and said I would rather listen to some music and catch up on the day's events. He shook his head OK, then smiled and told me I looked beautiful. I replied by telling him that he did, too. I could tell that he had no idea what I was up to. I began to get a little nervous, but even more excited. When he heard the song start, he looked up at me with a puzzled expression. Stage fright made me hesitate, but I really wanted to do this, and I couldn't believe how excited I was. As the music started, I slowly began to move my right hand up my left arm, across my shoulder, stopping my fingers just at the middle of my neck. For the first few moments I was afraid to lift my eyes to his. Finally I gathered the courage. The way he was staring at me, I knew then that I didn't have to worry. The look on his face said everything. As my hand slid down from my neck and disappeared under my blouse...his mouth couldn't have been open any wider."

As you can see, Maddy's synopsis wasn't all that short, but it gives you an example of what you are to do.

Often you'll be able to remember more details as you are writing down your recollection. You are attempting to re-create a clear, specific image of the episode. Now it's your turn.

SOUND SNAPSHOT FORM 1

Sound Focus:

Short Synopsis:

After you have finished your synopsis, put it aside for a while and focus your energy on something unrelated to Solid Therapy. Then, when you begin again, go over your story to see if you can recall any new details that can be added before proceeding.

Now you are to think about the event itself and narrow your recollection to one or two scenes that come to mind when you first think about the episode. Define the scene in terms of a snapshot. I will not elaborate on how to accomplish this. You should be very familiar with this procedure by now.

SOUND (SONG) SNAPSHOT RECOLLECTION FORM 1

Sound Focus:

____

____

Focal Item:

____

____

Short Snapshot Description:

____

____

____

____

____

____

____

____

After you have become aware of your initial picture and have written a short description of your snapshot, we will be almost ready to begin your lessons. Whereas before you were to pick out a Focal Item from your snapshot and use it as an initial focus for each lesson, for these lessons you will use the song or sound itself to initiate your recollection and eventually to reconstruct your snapshot.

Now we will outline how the next lessons are to proceed. Let us assume that you have chosen a song as your initiator. In each lesson you are to use your player to listen to the song. For now, do not play the entire song. Play only fifteen to thirty seconds of it. Then shift your attention to your Focal Item and begin to reconstruct your snapshot mentally. For an example, I have chosen the case study of a patient named Leslie.

CASE STUDY OF LESLIE

Song: *Sunday Morning Here with You* by Michael Franks.
Whenever Leslie heard that song, a particular image always came to mind. It was the image of an actual episode in her life. And for her lesson she described that image as if it were a snapshot:

"My bedroom on Brier; Michael Franks tapes were playing on the stereo in the other room. It was a cold Sunday morning in December. As you walk into the bedroom, the wall on the left is covered with two large sliding closet doors. The furniture is modern deco: two shiny black dressers, a nightstand, and matching headboard. A large black and gold-plated mirror across from the bed hanging over one of the dressers. On the dresser is a modern metal sculpture, a flat band that comes to a point at each end. The bed is queen-sized, with a dark gray comforter.

"Two thin, black metal floor lamps with inverted metal shades sit at each side of the bed. The wall to the left side of the bed is nothing but two large windows, which have both gray metal blinds and dark gray curtains. There is also a very large (six foot) ficus tree in the corner across from the bed. And a black easel with a painting of me on it. The blinds are partly open; sunlight is peeking through. My boyfriend is on the bed, wearing a mussed-up white dress shirt, left over from our night out, hanging open in the front with the sleeves rolled up. He also is wearing light gray cotton boxer shorts. He has on his brown thin-rimmed glasses, that he doesn't wear too often, but that I like a lot.

"He is lying on his side reading the paper, which is spread out all over the bed and the floor. Next to him on the bed is a white tray with a pot of tea, one cup, a plate of toast, and orange marmalade. I was wearing a very pretty, loosely fitted, white cotton teddy. There was no room on the bed for me, so I had several pillows fluffed up against the closet doors, and my butt was planted in the middle of them. I had one leg bent and the other stretched out and touching the side of the bed. My cup of tea was at my side as I took turns looking at my favorite sections of the paper and my boyfriend."

Leslie had chosen the white Irish china teapot as her Focal Item. To begin, she listened to the Michael Franks song for thirty seconds—long enough to get the song in her head. She then concentrated on her Focal Item—the teapot. After visualizing a clear image, she mentally reconstructed her snapshot. That is how Leslie did each lesson for the next two days.

Now it's your turn. On the form that follows write anything that stands out to you about your chosen event and anything new that you may have remembered, and then stop. This will conclude one lesson.

SOUND (SONG) SNAPSHOT RECOLLECTION FORM 2

Sound Focus:

Focal Item:

Short Recollection:

After you have completed this part of the lesson, you are ready for the next step. You no doubt are familiar with music videos on TV. They include both a song and a visual "story." Thus, music videos are not unlike your own experiences with certain songs and related events. Hearing and seeing create a very strong bond. That is, thinking of one causes you to think of the other. Hearing the song will almost always elicit the images of the video, and seeing the video will almost always elicit a recollection of the song. You do pretty much the same thing every day when you hear songs that cause you to remember something or someone. Usually the only difference is that your remembrance may not be as strongly connected because it lacks reinforcement. If the connection is not reinforced, as time goes by an increasing number of details eventually fade from your memory. This lessens the ability of a particular song to elicit a particular recollection.

Music videos are reinforced—viewed and listened to over and over—resulting in a strong association between the song and the visual image. Thus, someone who hears a particular song can easily associate it with its video. We are going to reinforce the associations of your own "music videos."

For this next series of lessons you need to be familiar with how to turn your snapshot into a dynamic movie. If you have forgotten part of this procedure, go back over Chapter Six before proceeding.

Each lesson should be performed in this manner: Begin by listening to your chosen song all the way through. However, instead of waiting until the song is over to begin your recollection and reconstruction, begin while the song is playing. First visualize your Focal Item, and then mentally reconstruct your snapshot. However, for now do not spend as much time on your reconstruction. By now you should be familiar enough with your reconstruction from previous lessons. Instead, devote most of your time to the actual recollection of the event. Remember that, just as before, after you have reconstructed your initial picture, treat it as if it were the opening scene in a movie. Then turn the movie on and watch it. Let your recollection of the event begin from that initial picture, allowing the movie to proceed from there.

SOUND (SONG) SNAPSHOT RECOLLECTION FORM 3

Sound Focus:

____

____

Focal Item:

____

____

Snapshot Recollection:

____

____

____

____

____

Items forgotten or not included during your recollection:

____

____

____

____

New items remembered during your recollection:

We'll continue with our case study of Leslie to illustrate how these lessons should be completed. Leslie began each lesson by turning on the song she had chosen. She would listen to it for several seconds before visualizing her Focal Item: the white teapot. At this point she did not turn off the player, but instead proceeded to reconstruct her snapshot quickly as the song played. Leslie then remembered the tray, her boyfriend, the bed covered with the Sunday paper. After she completed her mental image, she turned on her "movie." She allowed her snapshot to be the opening scene of her "movie" and continued with the story from there:

> "He looked so cute…I got a little excited. I wanted to get close to him, but I couldn't because the bed was covered with papers. So I climbed on the bed and pushed them all off. He hadn't eaten his toast yet, and when I jumped on the bed, I almost knocked everything over. He didn't get mad or anything; he just looked at me and laughed. I let one of the straps of my teddy slip off my shoulder…then took two of my fingers and put it in the marmalade. I glanced down and looked at my chest, then nudged the white, lacy cotton teddy lower until one breast was completely exposed. I asked him if he was hungry, staring right into his eyes. I wanted to see his face, his reaction as I took my orange-covered sticky fingers and spread the marmalade over my chest."

Using the forms below and in the Workbook Section, do one ten-minute lesson set, made up of one to two lessons, three times a day—morning, afternoon, and evening—for a total minimum of thirty minutes a day. Spend three days on each song before you repeat the entire series using a different song or sound as your generative focus. Then rest one day.

The volume at which your song is played is important. If it is played too loudly, it will distract you from recollecting your story. Just as when you're in your car and turn the volume of the radio way up, the decibel level saturates your conscious thoughts, making it virtually impossible for you to concentrate on anything else. Your song should be loud enough to be recognizable yet soft enough not to distract your thoughts. Here is what you are expected to complete in this part of your therapy.

First lesson series: (Use only one song/sound.)

A ten-minute lesson set, made up of one to two lessons, done three times a day—morning, afternoon, and evening—for a total minimum of thirty minutes a day for three days. Rest one day.

Second lesson series: (Use a minimum of five songs/sounds.)

A ten-minute lesson set, made up of one to two lessons, done three times a day—morning, afternoon, and evening—for a total minimum of thirty minutes a day, spending three days on each song. Rest one day.

SOUND (SONG) THERAPY LESSON FORM

Lesson 1 (Morning)

Items forgotten or not included during your recollection:

1. ______________________________

____

____

____

____

2. ______________________________

____

____

____

____

3. ______________________________

____

____

____

____

New items remembered during your recollection:

1. ______________________________

____

____

____

2.

3.

Lesson 2
Items forgotten or not included during your recollection:

1.

2.

3.

New items remembered during your recollection:

1. ______________________________

____

____

____

____

2. ______________________________

____

____

____

____

____

3. ______________________________

____

____

____

____

SOUND (SONG) THERAPY LESSON FORM

Lesson 1 (Afternoon)

Items forgotten or not included during your recollection:

1. ______________________________

____

____

____

____

____

____

2.

3.

New items remembered during your recollection:

1.

2.

3.

Lesson 2
Items forgotten or not included during your recollection:

1.

2

3.

New items remembered during your recollection:

1.

2.

3.

SOUND (SONG) THERAPY LESSON FORM

Lesson 1 (Evening)

Items forgotten or not included during your recollection:

1.

2.

3.

New items remembered during your recollection:

1.

2.

3.

Lesson 2
Items forgotten or not included during your recollection:

1.

2.

3.

New items remembered during your recollection:

1.

2.

3.

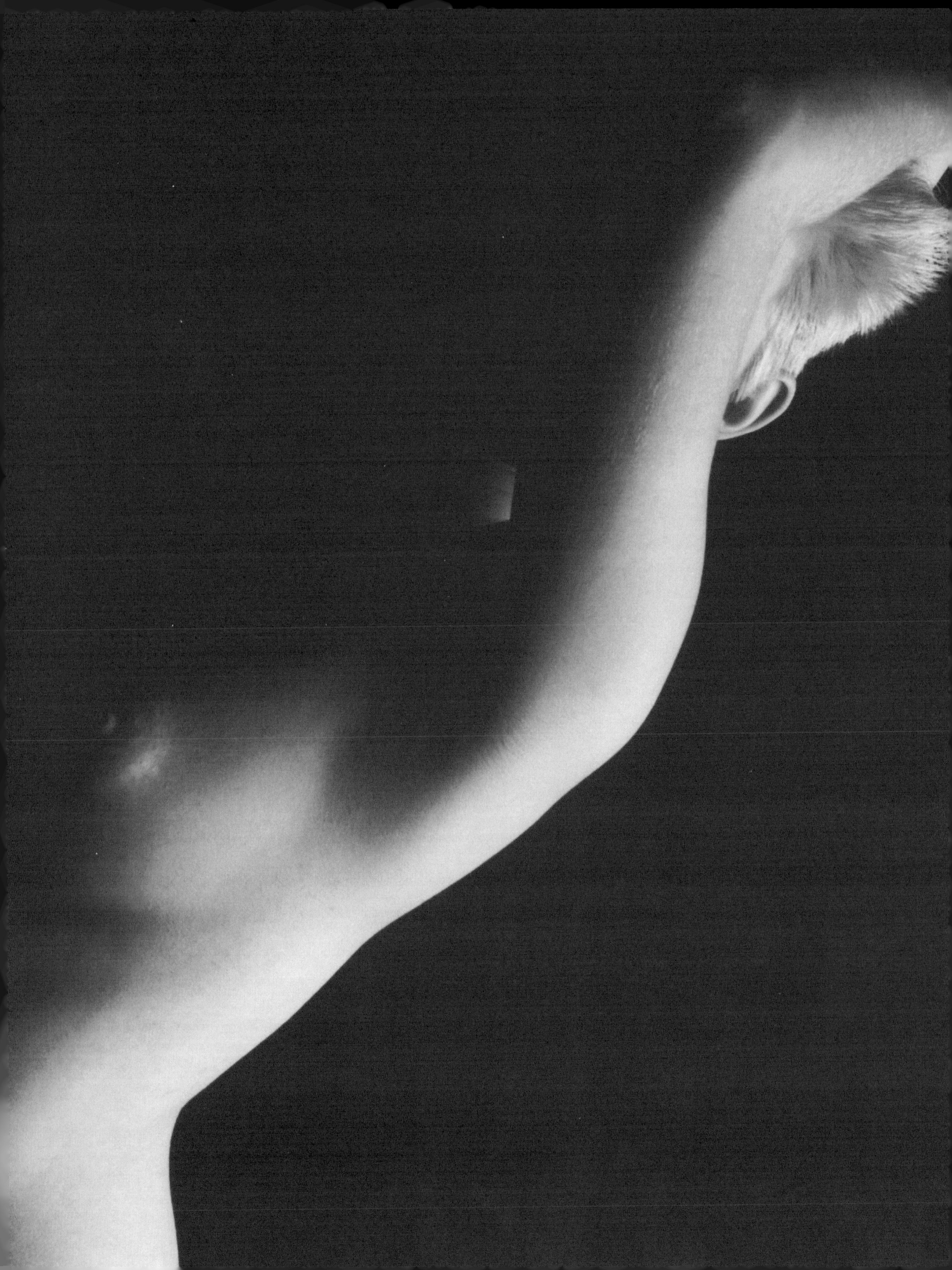

10

Chapter Ten

One More Time

Let me leave you with two illustrations of the difference that Solid Therapy can make in a couple's life. Penny, one of my first patients, found herself in a situation that seemed hopeless. "I'm a total failure at sex," she told me again and again. "I'm embarrassed to think about it ahead of time, and once we're in bed, it takes me just about half the night to feel sexy, if I ever do. Poor Rob [her boyfriend] works evenings, and our time together is so limited! So you can see where our love life is heading."

Rob also expressed some disappointment in their sex life, although he loved Penny and gave no indication that he would give up on their relationship. "She's great when she gets going," he joked, "but she so rarely gets going." She tried to laugh about it, but Penny's tightly clenched hands told me how serious the problem really was. She was devastated and said that she often felt unsexy and unfeminine. She had even gained ten pounds "out of frustration."

When I asked Penny to talk to me about something that she thought was sexy, she blushed and rambled on about a movie that she had seen on television. "The hero, he sort of started to make out with a girl in the swimming pool...," she faltered. "See—I still can't do it!"

Penny didn't think she would ever be able to bridge the libido gap that separated Rob and herself. However, she wasn't quite resigned to a life without sexual pleasure, and so, mostly for Rob's sake, she tried Solid Therapy. Rob didn't push the matter, but I could see how eager he was for the system to work.

One day, after eight weeks of Solid Therapy, Penny bounced into my office positively glowing. Her posture was different, her hairstyle was different. And most impressive, her face was different—she was smiling broadly. "It works, *it works*!" she almost sang. "Ask me about sex again," she grinned.

I did, and she spent the next half hour telling me about all the mental techniques that she had learned that allowed her to turn on "the sex faucet," as she called it.

"Rob is switching to days," she said, "although to tell you the truth, it doesn't make any difference to us anymore whether we make love days or nights. It's there…I can have a great time whenever I want."

She paused for a breath. "When I first came here, I didn't believe I'd ever say this, but I feel so alive and sexy!" Obviously her self-confidence had skyrocketed! And remember April and Ryan, whom we met in Chapter Two? Recently April told me: "Ryan still gets a kick out of the change in me! Of course, there are times when I don't want any sex at all, and he respects that. But, boy, I know which mental buttons to push now when I want to get in the mood…I initiate our lovemaking a lot more…I never imagined sex could be this thrilling."

Penny and April succeeded with Solid Therapy for two reasons. First, they were sensitive enough to realize that the problem in their relationships might lie partially with them and that it needed to be addressed. And second, they were willing to make the effort to help themselves and ultimately their relationships.

Another important factor in Penny's and April's success was their attention to details. Let me tell you a little secret about details. Even though I have emphasized details throughout this book, I haven't explained their importance until now for a reason: I have found that too often when patients were told of the importance of details at the start of Solid Therapy, some of them became lazy and failed to push their memory and imagination, finishing just the minimum amount of lessons. Many times, after selecting a Focal Item they would begin a lesson without pressing their memory, thereby missing the most important part of their therapy. Just as your muscles will not grow stronger without the proper exercise, so also your sensual "muscles" need their proper exercise. So please don't cut corners with details. Remember that you are doing this therapy to heighten your sexual awareness and responsiveness so that you and your partner can enjoy a truly healthy, energetic sex life.

Details are crucial to your success because the more details you see that remind you of something sexual, the more you *think* about something sexual. So many people, things, and events in our lives could serve as erotic stimuli, but we either *neglect* or *choose not to recognize* them.

Our goal has been not only to help you to rediscover the sexual pleasure hiding within ordinary things and events in your life, but also to help you to develop strong associations between those things and events and your libido. Ultimately, this will let you widen your sensitivity to once-neutral elements, allowing you to activate your sensual "taste buds" easily. Consequently, erotic associations will lead to erotic thoughts, similar to the way that the smell of chocolate makes your mouth water and visions of creamy chocolate candy flash before your mind's eye.

Don't feel overwhelmed by all the work that I am asking you to do. It takes some time and effort. But it pays off. Remember that no one is going to grade your lessons. There are no wrong answers, only answers that will help to brighten your life.

If you'd like to read more about the topics we've covered in this book, I recommend: *Child Development and Personality* by Paul Henry Mussen; *The Psychology of Gender,* edited by Robert J. Sternberg and Anne E. Beal; *The Question of Sex Differences—Psychological, Cultural, and Biological Issues* by Katherine Blick Hoyenga and Kermit T. Hoyenga; *Sexual Images of the Self—The Psychology of Erotic Sensations and Illusions* by Seymour Fisher; *and Peer Relationships in Child Development,* edited by Thomas J. Berndt and Gary W. Ladd.

I remain interested in your progress with Solid Therapy. After you've had time to read the book carefully, to do the lessons, and to master Solid Therapy, you could do me—and women like yourself—a favor by answering the following questions and mailing your answers to me at:

Michael. P. Bonaventura, M.D.
P.O. Box 1542
Evanston, IL 60204-1542

Please be as honest and as detailed as you can. You need not include your name and address, of course, unless you'd like a response.

1. In what way(s) has Solid Therapy made sex better for you?
2. Do you find sex easier to think about now? In what ways?
3. Do you feel that you are more in control of sex after Solid Therapy? If so, in what ways?
4. Has your sexual partner(s) noticed less inhibition on your part? If so, how has this improved your relationship(s)?
5. Did you find the book's exercises enjoyable? Do you still focus on "snapshots" at odd times during the day?
6. Which exercise "snapshot" was most useful to you? Why?
7. What did you find most useful about Solid Therapy? Why?
8. What did you find least useful about Solid Therapy? Why?
9. Would you recommend this book to others? Why?
10. If you were in my office right now, what would you say to me, good or bad, about this book and Solid Therapy? Be candid.

In closing, I would like to say how much I genuinely admire you for being open enough to try something new and for having the courage to tackle such a personal subject. Just keep in mind that you have a right to enjoy sex on your own terms, when and where you want it. You have the right to enjoy sex as much as men do!

I've enjoyed sharing Solid Therapy with you, and I am confident that you will do well with it. Good luck. And have fun. After all, that's what sex is all about!

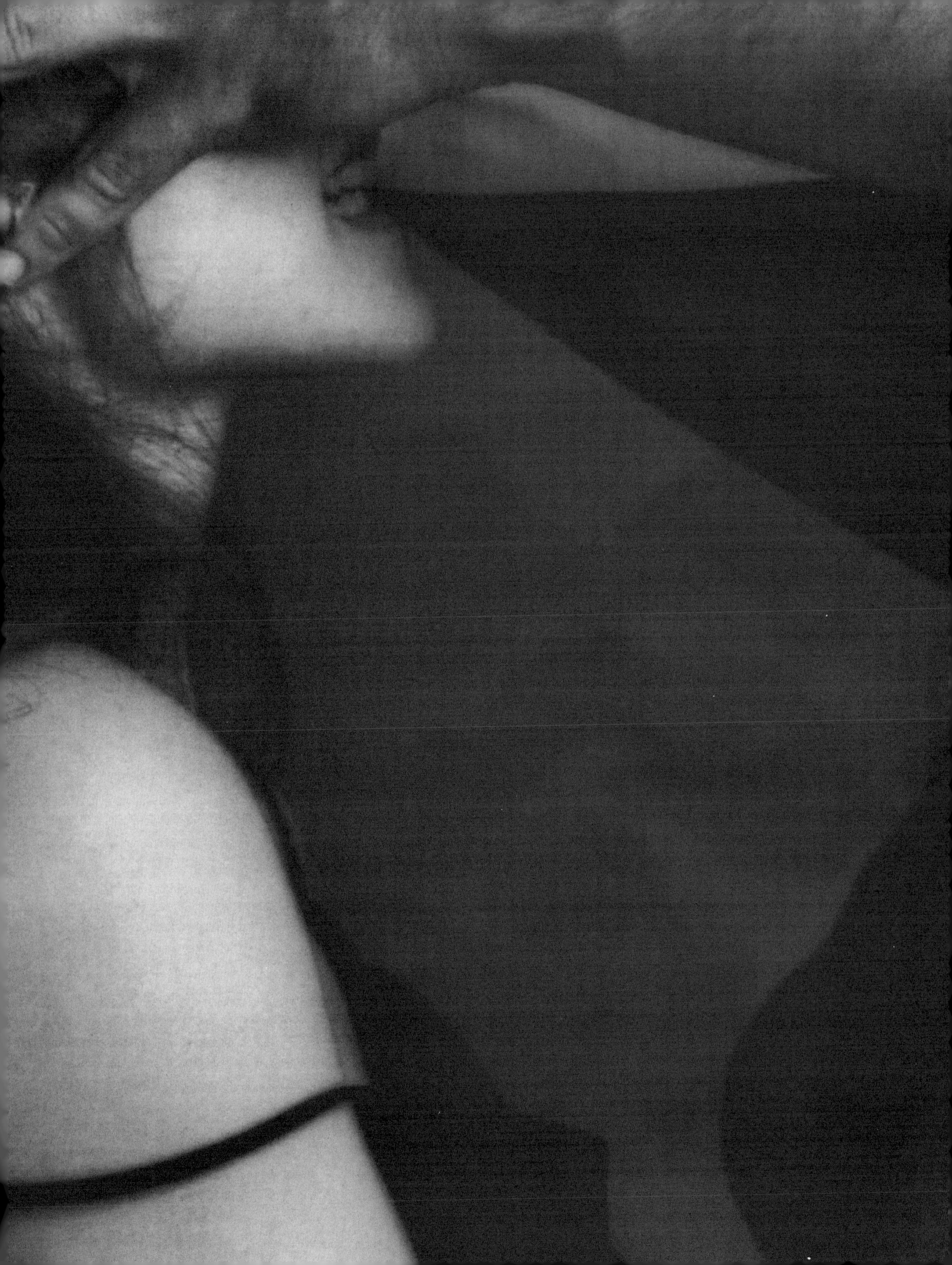

Workbook Section

QUESTIONNAIRE FORMS

FIRST LIST OF AROUSING SUBJECTS

Directions: 1. Review Chapters Four and Five before completing this form.
Question: What subjects— persons, places, things, and events— do you find arousing?

List your answers in the spaces provided.

1. ______________________________

____

____

____

____

2. ______________________________

____

____

____

____

3. ______________________________

____

____

____

____

4. ______________________________

____

____

____

____

____

5. ______________________________

____

____

____

____

6. ______________________________

____

____

____

____

7. ______________________________

____

____

____

8. ______________________________

____

____

____

SECOND LIST OF AROUSING SUBJECTS

Directions:

1. Review Chapters Four through Six before beginning.
2. After going over your thoughts and the list you just made, narrow your arousing subjects to six that you wish to use for your future lessons. Order your responses from most erotic to least erotic.
3. Write down your responses using only a few words to identify each one. You will refer to them later.

1. ______________________________

____

2.

3.

4.

5.

6.

MOST AROUSING SUBJECT

Directions: Now from your second list, choose the subject that you find most arousing to begin your lessons with.

SNAPSHOT RECOLLECTION FORMS

Directions:

1. Review Chapters Four through Six before you begin.
2. Describe the picture that first comes to your mind when you think of the subject that you chose. Describe it as if you were describing a "snapshot."
3. Fill in with as much detail as you can.
4. Take your time and, most important, do not cut short your recollection.

INITIAL SNAPSHOT RECOLLECTION FORM

SECOND SNAPSHOT RECOLLECTION FORM

Directions:

1. Review Chapters Four through Six before beginning.
2. Complete the Initial Snapshot Recollection Form before attempting this form.
3. Choose at least one Focal Item before completing this form.
4. Take your time and try not to omit any details.

Focal Items:

1. ______
2. ______
3. ______
4. ______

Second Snapshot Recollection:

FINAL SNAPSHOT RECOLLECTION FORM

Directions:

1. Review Chapters Four through Six before beginning.
2. Complete the Initial and Second Snapshot Recollection Forms first.
3. Complete this form as outlined in Chapter Six.
4. Take your time and try not to cut short your recollection.

Focal Items:

1. ____________________

2. ____________________

Final Snapshot Recollection:

Items forgotten or not included during your recollection:

1.

2.

3.

New items remembered during your recollection:

1.

2.

3.

- These snapshot recollection lessons are printed twice to give you plenty of space.

Directions: Review Chapter Six before completing these lessons.

SNAPSHOT RECOLLECTION FORM
Lesson 1 (Morning)
Items forgotten or not included during your recollection:

1. ______

2. ______

3. ______

New items remembered during your recollection:

1. ______

2.

3.

Lesson 2
Items forgotten or not included during your recollection:

1.

2.

3.

New items remembered during your recollection:

1. ______

2. ______

3. ______

Lesson 3
Items forgotten or not included during your recollection:

1. ______

2. ______

3.

New items remembered during your recollection:

1.

2.

3.

Lesson 4
Items forgotten or not included during your recollection:

1.

2.

3.

New items remembered during your recollection:

1.

2.

3.

SNAPSHOT RECOLLECTION FORM

Lesson 1 (Afternoon)

Items forgotten or not included during your recollection:

1. ______________________________

2. ______________________________

3. ______________________________

New items remembered during your recollection:

1. ______________________________

2. ______________________________

3.

Lesson 2
Items forgotten or not included during your recollection:

1.

2.

3.

New items remembered during your recollection:

1.

2.

3.

Lesson 3
Items forgotten or not included during your recollection:

1.

2.

3.

New items remembered during your recollection:

1.

2.

3.

Lesson 4

Items forgotten or not included during your recollection:

1.

2.

3.

New items remembered during your recollection:

1.

2.

3.

SNAPSHOT RECOLLECTION FORM

Lesson 1 (EVENING)

Items forgotten or not included during your recollection:

1.

2.

3.

New items remembered during your recollection:

1.

2.

3.

Lesson 2
Items forgotten or not included during your recollection:

1.

2.

3.

New items remembered during your recollection:

1.

2.

3.

Lesson 3
Items forgotten or not included during your recollection:

1.

2.

3.

New items remembered during your recollection:

1.

2.

3.

Lesson 4
Items forgotten or not included during your recollection:

1.

2.

3.

New items remembered during your recollection:

1.

2.

3.

FINAL MOVIE RECOLLECTION FORM
Lesson 1 (MORNING)
Items or feelings forgotten or not included during your movie recollection:

1. ______________________________

____

____

____

____

2. ______________________________

____

____

____

____

3. ______________________________

____

____

____

____

New items or feelings remembered during your movie recollection:

1. ______________________________

____

____

____

____

2. ______________________________

____

3.

Lesson 2

Items or feelings forgotten or not included during your movie recollection:

1.

2.

3.

New items or feelings remembered during your movie recollection:

1.

2.

3.

Lesson 3
Items or feelings forgotten or not included during your movie recollection:

1.

2.

3.

New items or feelings remembered during your movie recollection:

1.

2.

3.

Lesson 4

Items or feelings forgotten or not included during your movie recollection:

1.

2.

3.

New items or feelings remembered during your movie recollection:

1.

2.

3.

FINAL MOVIE RECOLLECTION FORM

Lesson 1 (Afternoon)

Items or feelings forgotten or not included during your movie recollection:

1. ______

2. ______

3. ______

New items or feelings remembered during your movie recollection:

1. ______

2. ______

3.

Lesson 2

Items or feelings forgotten or not included during your movie recollection:

1.

2.

3.

New items or feelings remembered during your movie recollection:

1.

2.

3.

Lesson 3

Items or feelings forgotten or not included during your movie recollection:

1.

2.

3.

New items or feelings remembered during your movie recollection:

1. ______________________________

____

____

____

____

2. ______________________________

____

____

____

____

3. ______________________________

____

____

____

____

Lesson 4

Items or feelings forgotten or not included during your movie recollection:

1. ______________________________

____

____

____

____

2. ______________________________

____

____

____

3.

New items or feelings remembered during your movie recollection:

1.

2.

3.

FINAL MOVIE RECOLLECTION FORM

Lesson 1 (EVENING)

Items or feelings forgotten or not included during your movie recollection:

1. ______

2. ______

3. ______

New items or feelings remembered during your movie recollection:

1. ______

2. ______

3.

Lesson 2

Items or feelings forgotten or not included during your movie recollection:

1.

2.

3.

New items or feelings remembered during your movie recollection:

1. ______________________________

2. ______________________________

3. ______________________________

Lesson 3

Items or feelings forgotten or not included during your movie recollection:

1. ______________________________

2. ______________________________

3.

New items or feelings remembered during your movie recollection:

1.

2.

3.

Lesson 4

Items or feelings forgotten or not included during your movie recollection:

1.

2.

3.

New items or feelings remembered during your movie recollection:

1.

2.

3.

VISUAL SUBSIDY SNAPSHOT RECOLLECTION FORMS

Directions:

1. Review Chapters Four through Six and Chapter Eight before beginning.

2. Describe your Visual Subsidy in the forms as directed in Chapter Eight.

Initial Visual Subsidy Snapshot Recollection

- When you have completed this form, continue to the next.

FINAL VISUAL SUBSIDY SNAPSHOT RECOLLECTION FORM

Lesson 1

Focal Item:

Recollection:

Like Items	Unlike Items	Missing Items

Lesson 2

Focal Item:

Recollection:

Like Items	Unlike Items	Missing Items

Lesson 3
Focal Item:

Recollection:

Like Items	Unlike Items	Missing Items

Lesson 4
Focal Item:

Recollection:

Like Items	Unlike Items	Missing Items

• The following forms are for one lesson series to accompany Chapter Nine. Before you complete them, review the chapter.

SOUND (SONG) THERAPY LESSON FORM
Lesson 1 (MORNING)
Items forgotten or not included during your recollection:

1. ______________________________

____

____

____

____

2. ______________________________

____

____

____

____

3. ______________________________

____

____

____

____

New items remembered during your recollection:

1. ______________________________

____

____

____

____

____

2.

3.

Lesson 2
Items forgotten or not included during your recollection:

1.

2.

3.

New items remembered during your recollection:

1. ____

2. ____

3. ____

SOUND (SONG) THERAPY LESSON FORM
Lesson 1 (Afternoon)
Items forgotten or not included during your recollection:

1. ____

2. ____

3.

New items remembered during your recollection:

1.

2.

3.

Lesson 2
Items forgotten or not included during your recollection:

1.

2.

3.

New items remembered during your recollection:

1.

2.

3.

SOUND (SONG) THERAPY LESSON FORM

Lesson 1 (Evening)

Items forgotten or not included during your recollection:

1. ______________________________

____

____

____

____

2. ______________________________

____

____

____

____

3. ______________________________

____

____

____

____

New items remembered during your recollection:

1. ______________________________

____

____

____

____

2. ______________________________

____

____

3.

Lesson 2
Items forgotten or not included during your recollection:

1.

2.

3.

New items remembered during your recollection:

1.

2.

3.

EXTRA SPACE FOR YOUR NOTES: